KIMIKO
DOES
CANCER

KIMIKO DOES CANCER

A Graphic Memoir

KIMIKO TOBIMATSU

ILLUSTRATED BY
KEET GENIZA

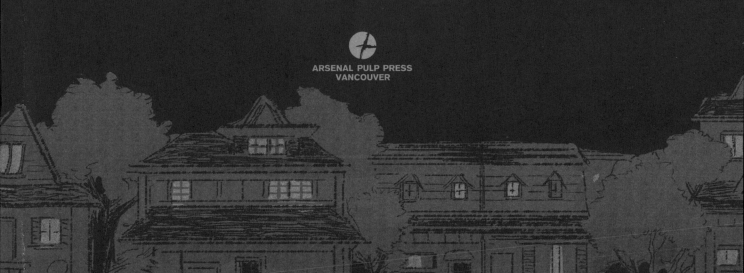

ARSENAL PULP PRESS
VANCOUVER

ARSENAL PULP PRESS
Suite 202 – 211 East Georgia St.
Vancouver, BC V6A 1Z6
Canada
arsenalpulp.com

The publisher gratefully acknowledges the support of the Canada Council for the Arts and the
British Columbia Arts Council for its publishing program, and the Government of Canada, and
the Government of British Columbia (through the Book Publishing Tax Credit Program), for its
publishing activities.

 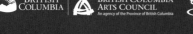

Arsenal Pulp Press acknowledges the xʷməθkʷəẏəm (Musqueam), Sḵwx̱wú7mesh (Squamish),
and səl̓ilwətaʔɬ (Tsleil-Waututh) Nations, custodians of the traditional, ancestral and unceded
territories where our office is located. We pay respect to their histories, traditions and continuous
living cultures and commit to accountability, respectful relations and friendship.

Cover illustrations by Keet Geniza
Cover design by Jazmin Welch
Edited by Shirarose Wilensky
Proofread by Alison Strobel

Printed and bound in Canada

Library and Archives Canada Cataloguing in Publication:
Title: Kimiko does cancer : a graphic memoir / Kimiko Tobimatsu ; illustrated by Keet Geniza.
Names: Tobimatsu, Kimiko, 1989– author. | Geniza, Keet, 1987– illustrator.
Identifiers: Canadiana (print) 2020021103X | Canadiana (ebook) 20200211080 |
  ISBN 9781551528199 (softcover) | ISBN 9781551528205 (HTML)
Subjects: LCSH: Tobimatsu, Kimiko, 1989-—Comic books, strips, etc. | LCSH: Tobimatsu,
  Kimiko, 1989-—Health—Comic books, strips, etc. | LCSH: Breast—Cancer—Patients—
  Canada—Biography—Comic books, strips, etc. | LCSH: Breast—Cancer—Comic books,
  strips, etc. | LCSH: Sexual minority women—Canada—Biography—Comic books, strips, etc. |
  LCSH: Racially mixed women—Canada—Biography—Comic books, strips, etc. |
  LCGFT: Autobiographical comics.
Classification: LCC RC280.B8 T63 2020 | DDC 362.19699/4490092—dc23

To our fellow sick queers.

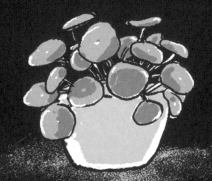

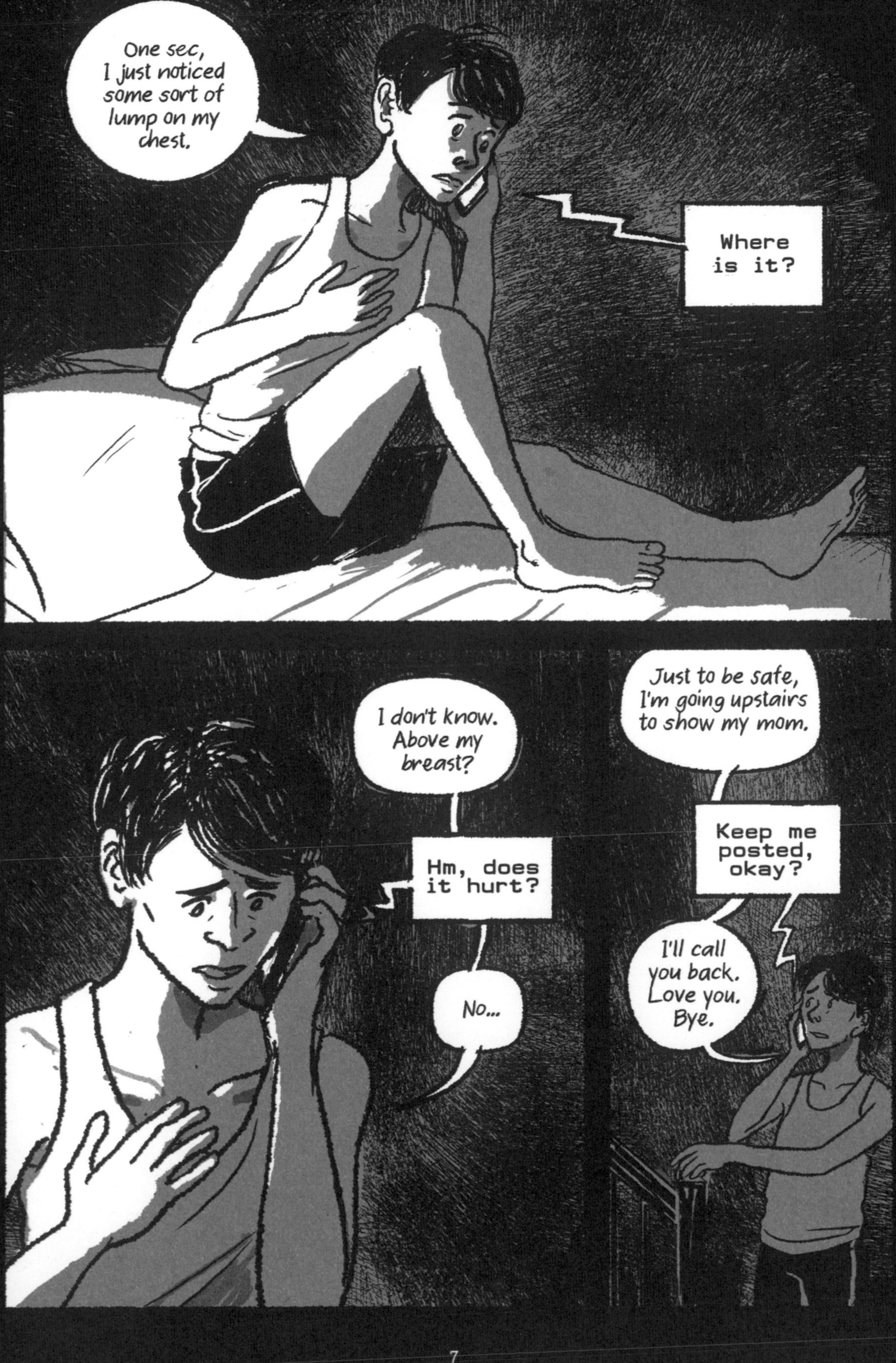
One sec, I just noticed some sort of lump on my chest.
Where is it?
I don't know. Above my breast?
Hm, does it hurt?
No...
Just to be safe, I'm going upstairs to show my mom.
Keep me posted, okay?
I'll call you back. Love you. Bye.

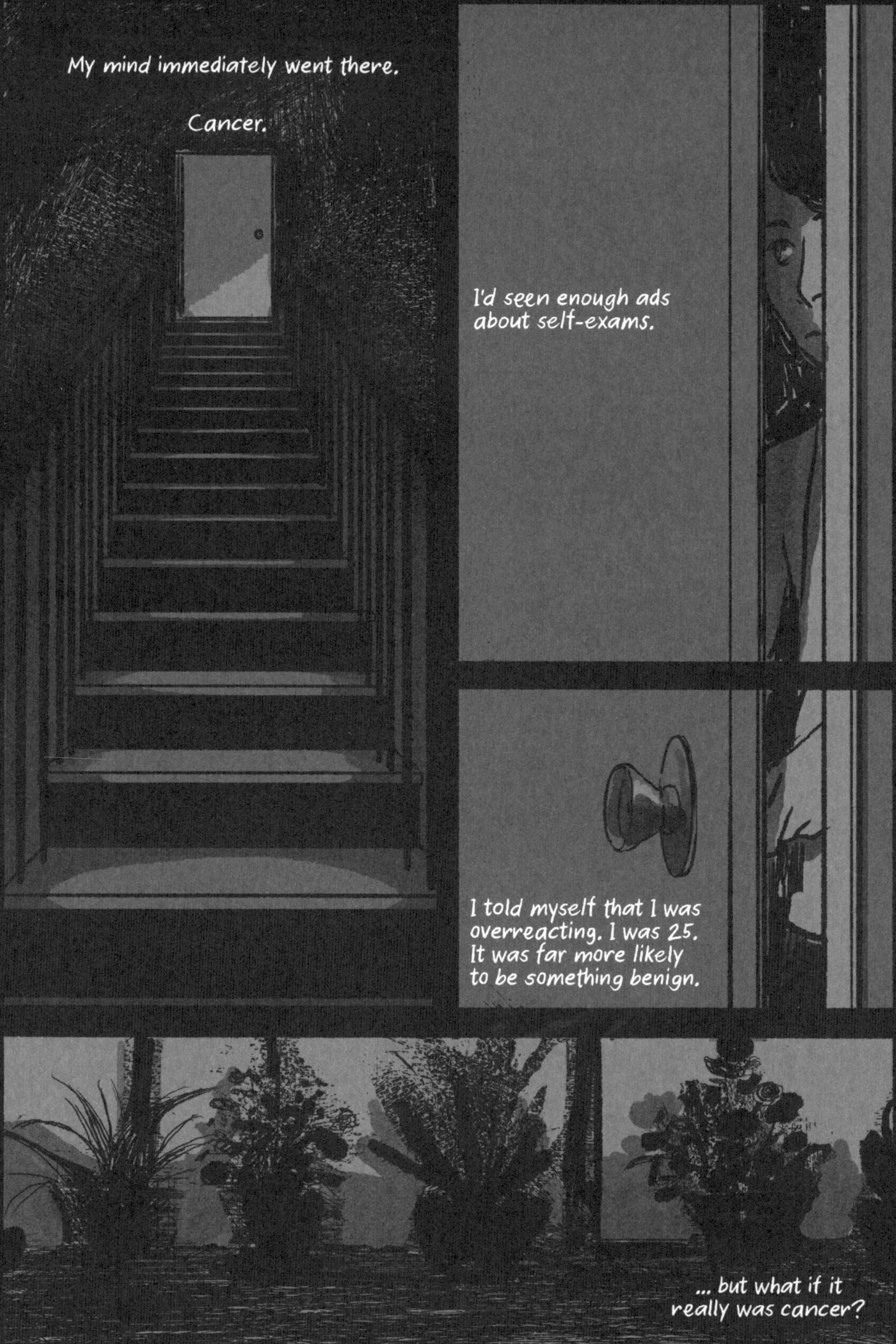
My mind immediately went there.
Cancer.
I'd seen enough ads about self-exams.
I told myself that I was overreacting. I was 25. It was far more likely to be something benign.
... but what if it really was cancer?

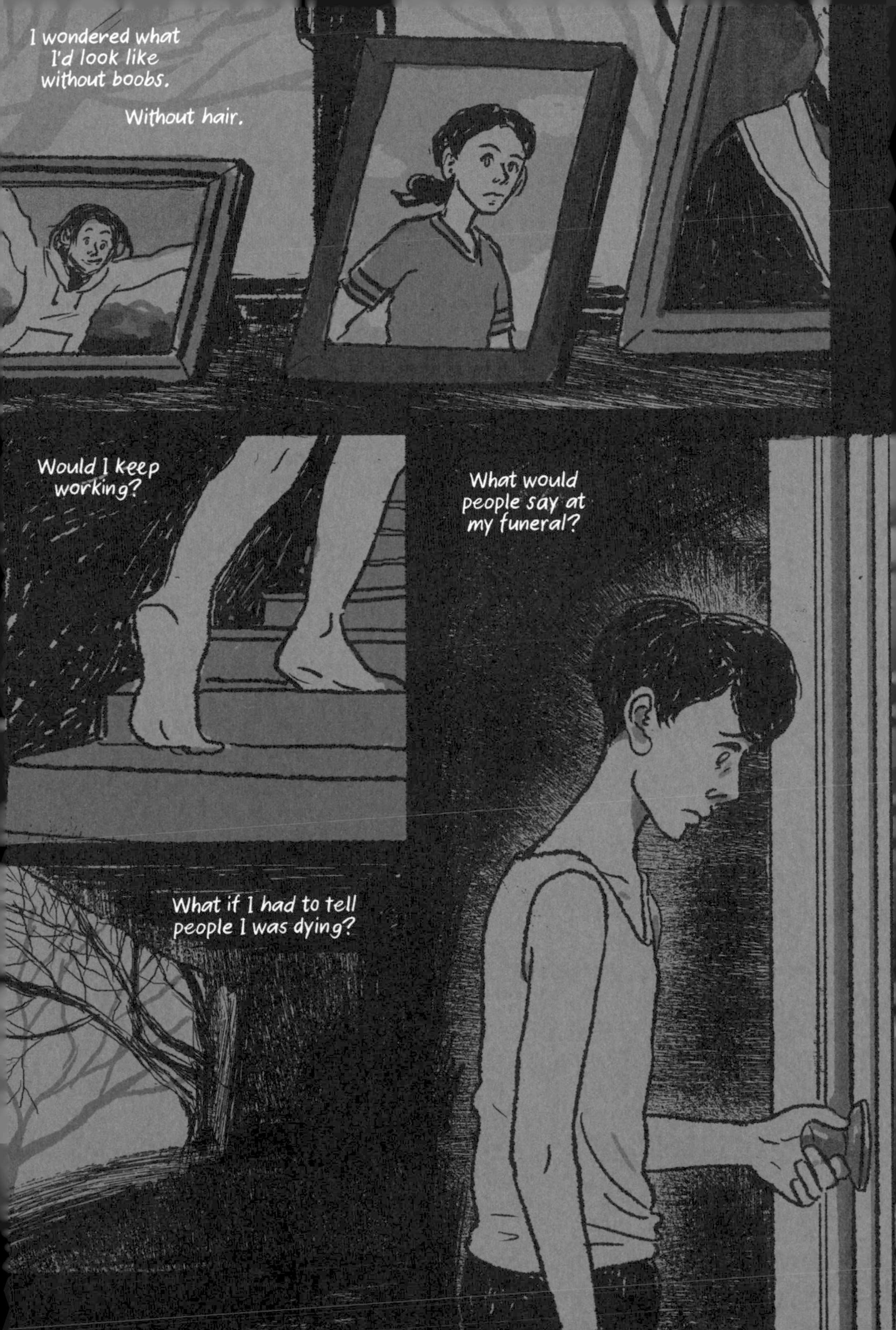
I wondered what I'd look like without boobs.
Without hair.
Would I keep working?
What would people say at my funeral?
What if I had to tell people I was dying?

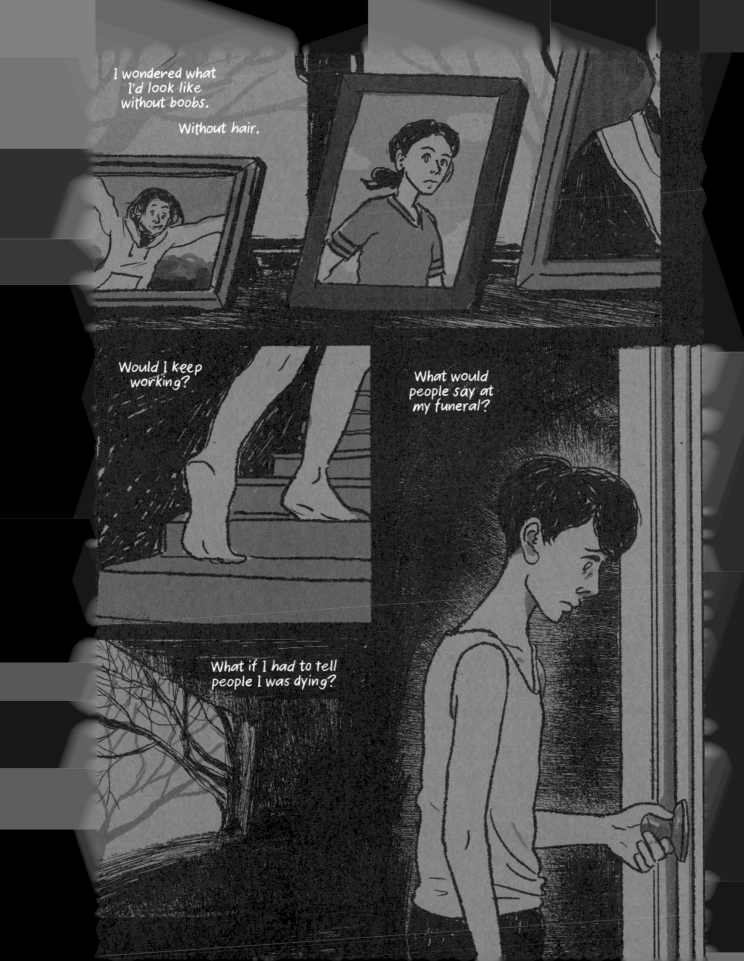

THE DIAGNOSIS

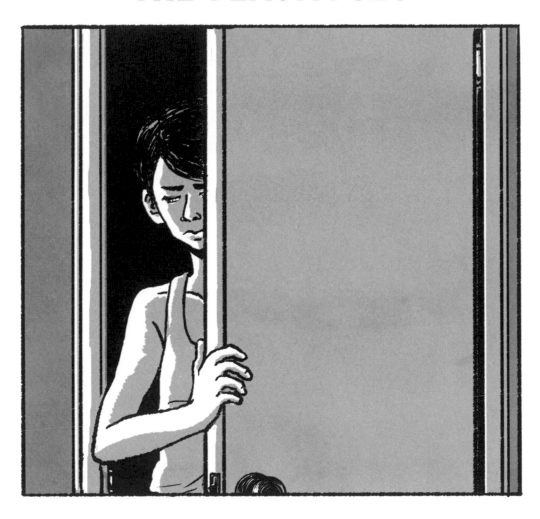

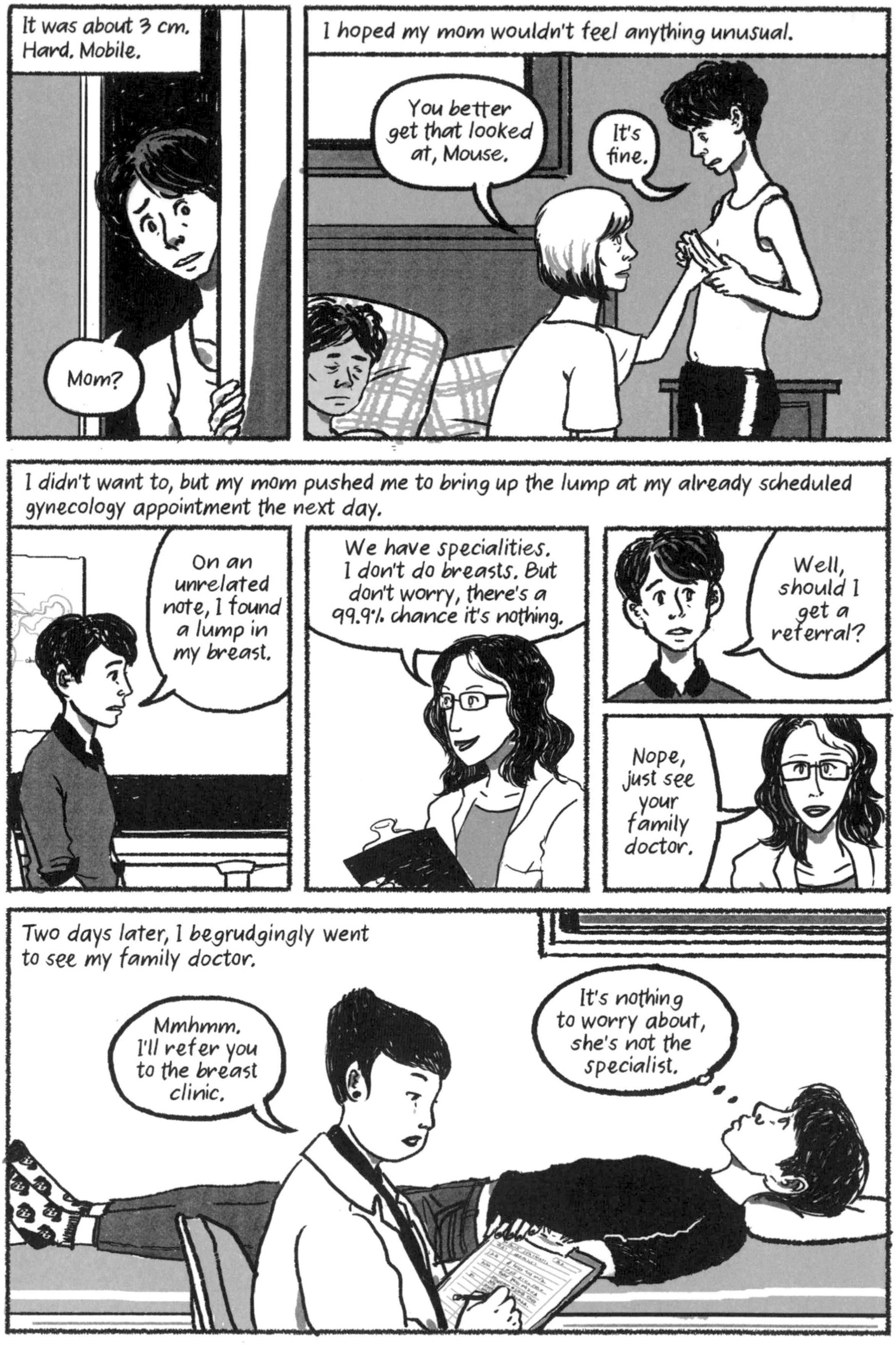
It was about 3 cm. Hard. Mobile.
Mom?
I hoped my mom wouldn't feel anything unusual.
You better get that looked at, Mouse.
It's fine.
I didn't want to, but my mom pushed me to bring up the lump at my already scheduled gynecology appointment the next day.
On an unrelated note, I found a lump in my breast.
We have specialities. I don't do breasts. But don't worry, there's a 99.9% chance it's nothing.
Well, should I get a referral?
Nope, just see your family doctor.
Two days later, I begrudgingly went to see my family doctor.
Mmhmm. I'll refer you to the breast clinic.
It's nothing to worry about, she's not the specialist.

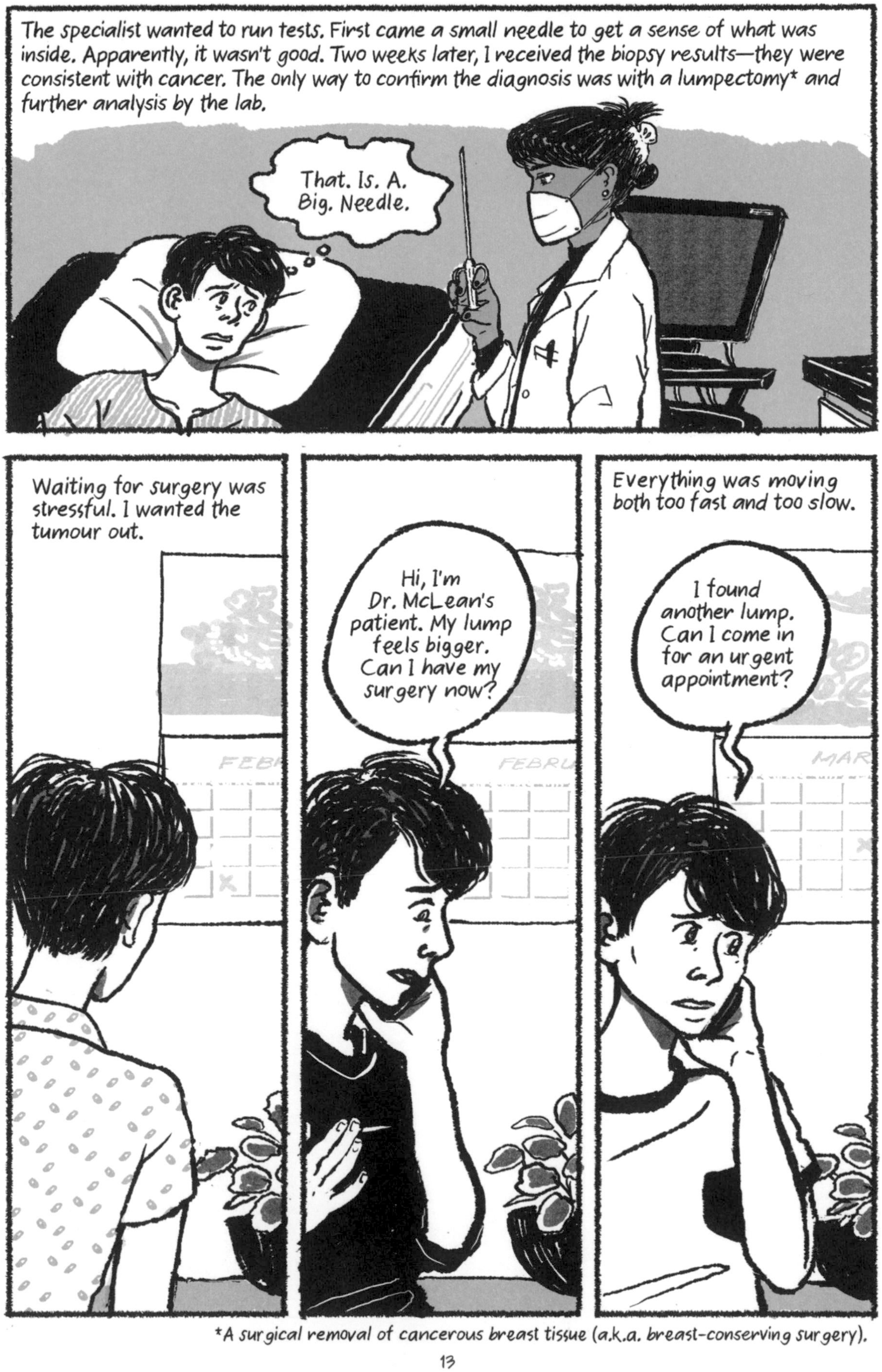
The specialist wanted to run tests. First came a small needle to get a sense of what was inside. Apparently, it wasn't good. Two weeks later, I received the biopsy results—they were consistent with cancer. The only way to confirm the diagnosis was with a lumpectomy* and further analysis by the lab.
That. Is. A. Big. Needle.
Waiting for surgery was stressful. I wanted the tumour out.
Hi, I'm Dr. McLean's patient. My lump feels bigger. Can I have my surgery now?
Everything was moving both too fast and too slow.
I found another lump. Can I come in for an urgent appointment?

*A surgical removal of cancerous breast tissue (a.k.a. breast-conserving surgery).

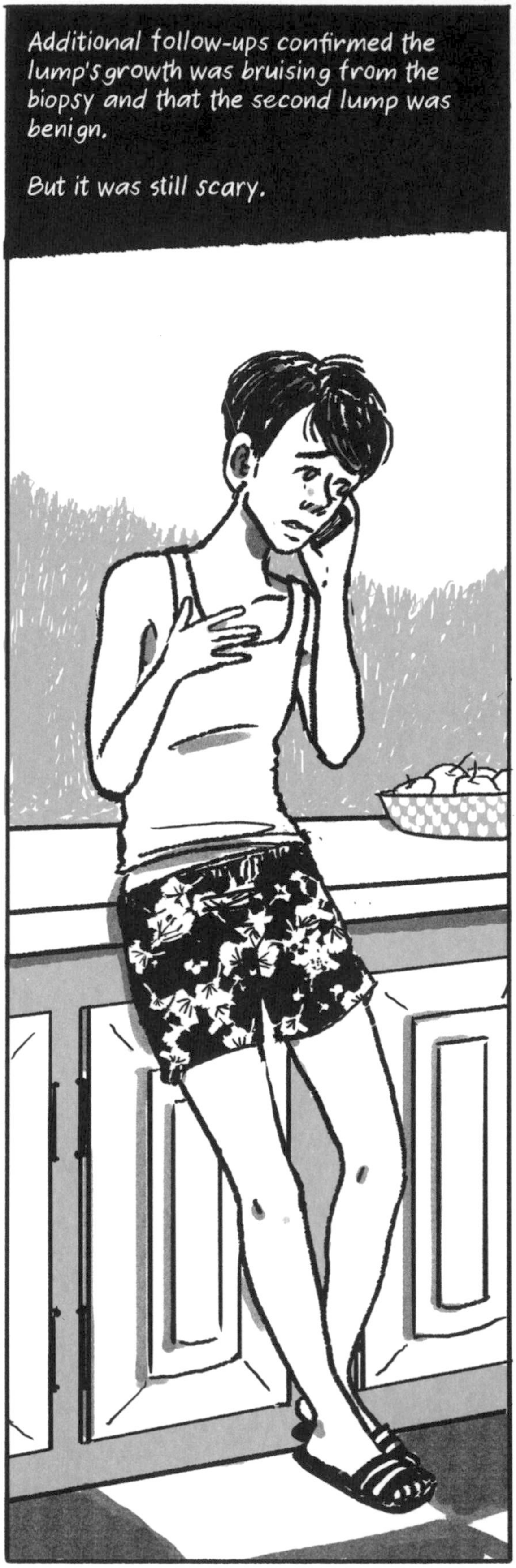
Additional follow-ups confirmed the lump's growth was bruising from the biopsy and that the second lump was benign.
But it was still scary.

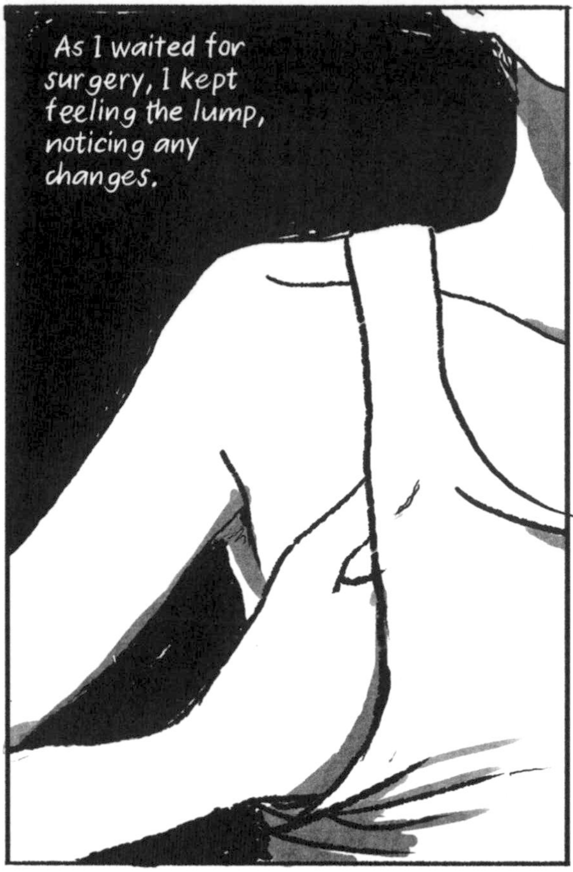
As I waited for surgery, I kept feeling the lump, noticing any changes.

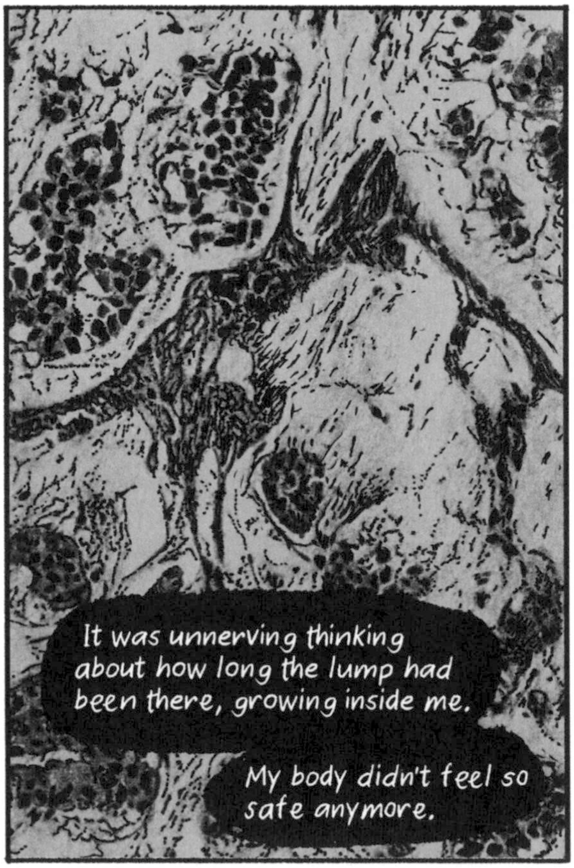
It was unnerving thinking about how long the lump had been there, growing inside me.
My body didn't feel so safe anymore.

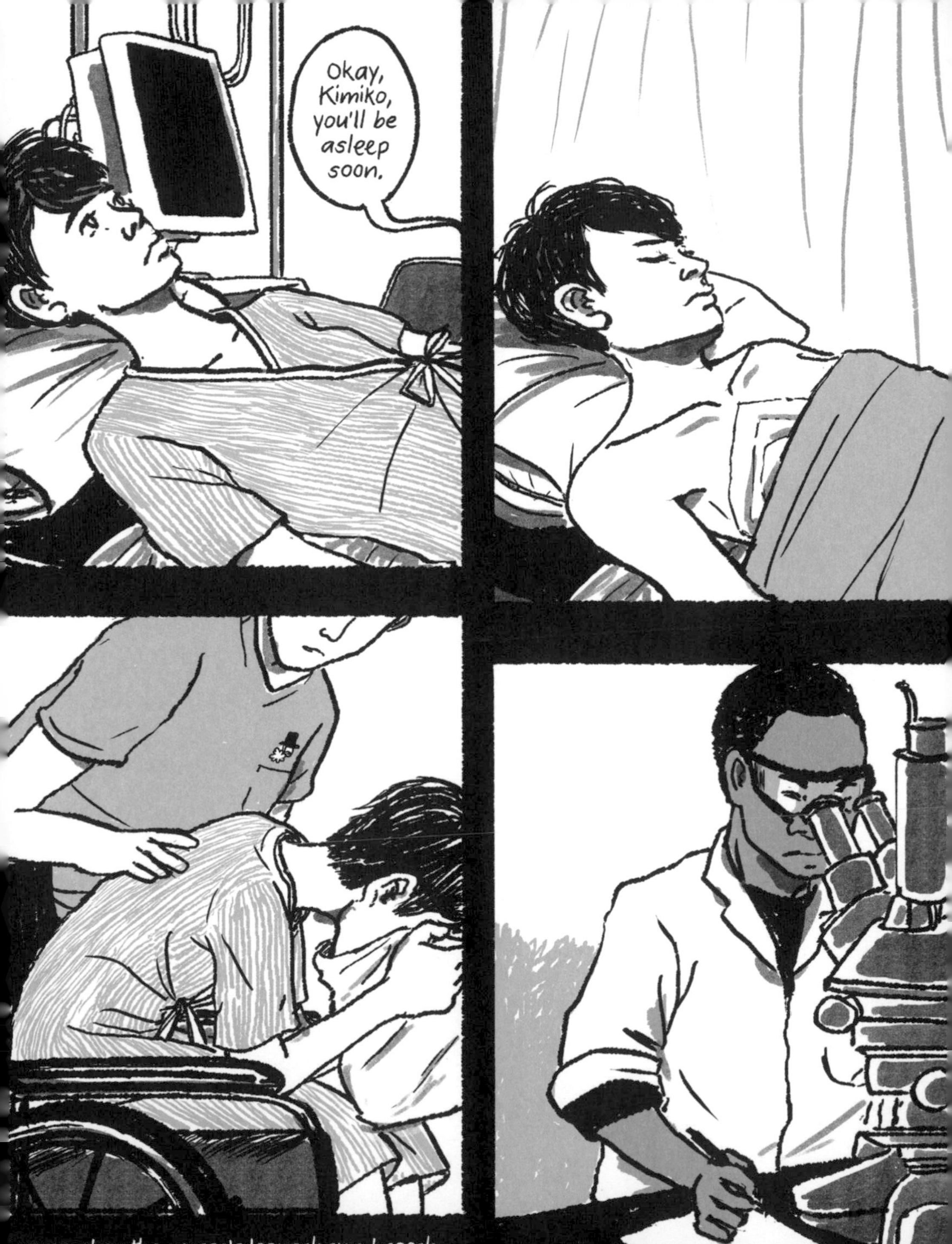
Okay, Kimiko, you'll be asleep soon.

remember the nurse's leprechaun brooch

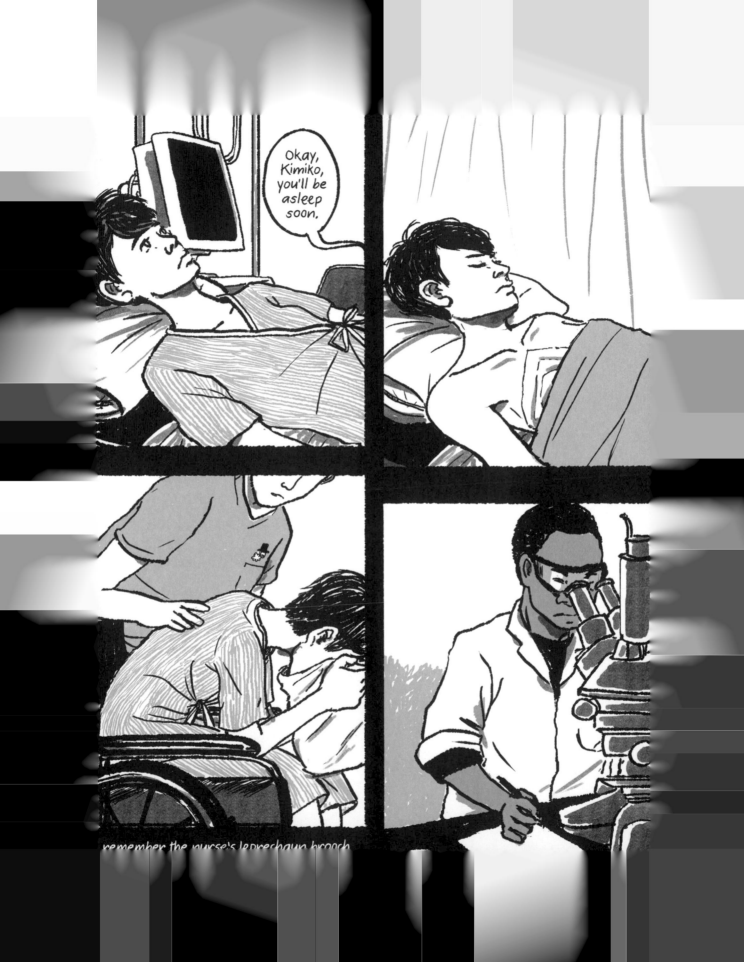

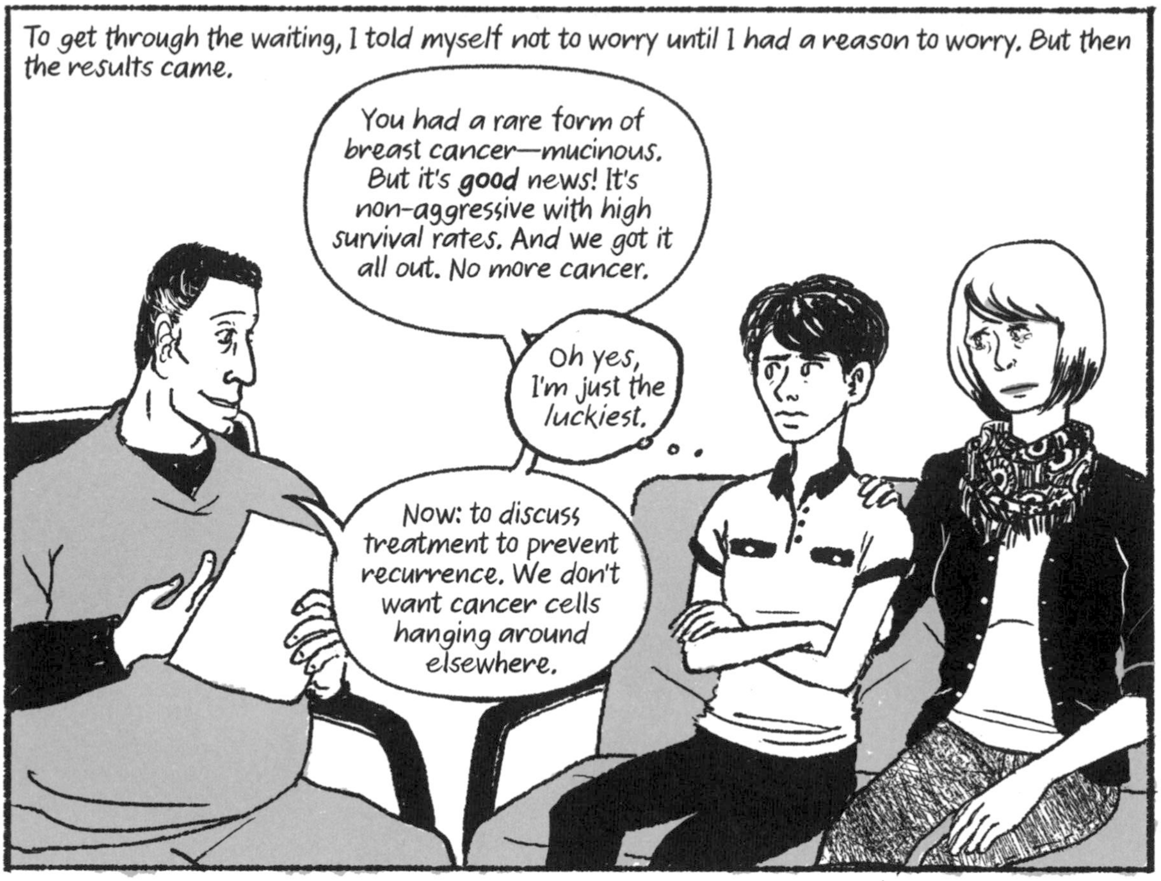
To get through the waiting, I told myself not to worry until I had a reason to worry. But then the results came.
You had a rare form of breast cancer—mucinous. But it's **good** news! It's non-aggressive with high survival rates. And we got it all out. No more cancer.
Oh yes, I'm just the luckiest.
Now: to discuss treatment to prevent recurrence. We don't want cancer cells hanging around elsewhere.

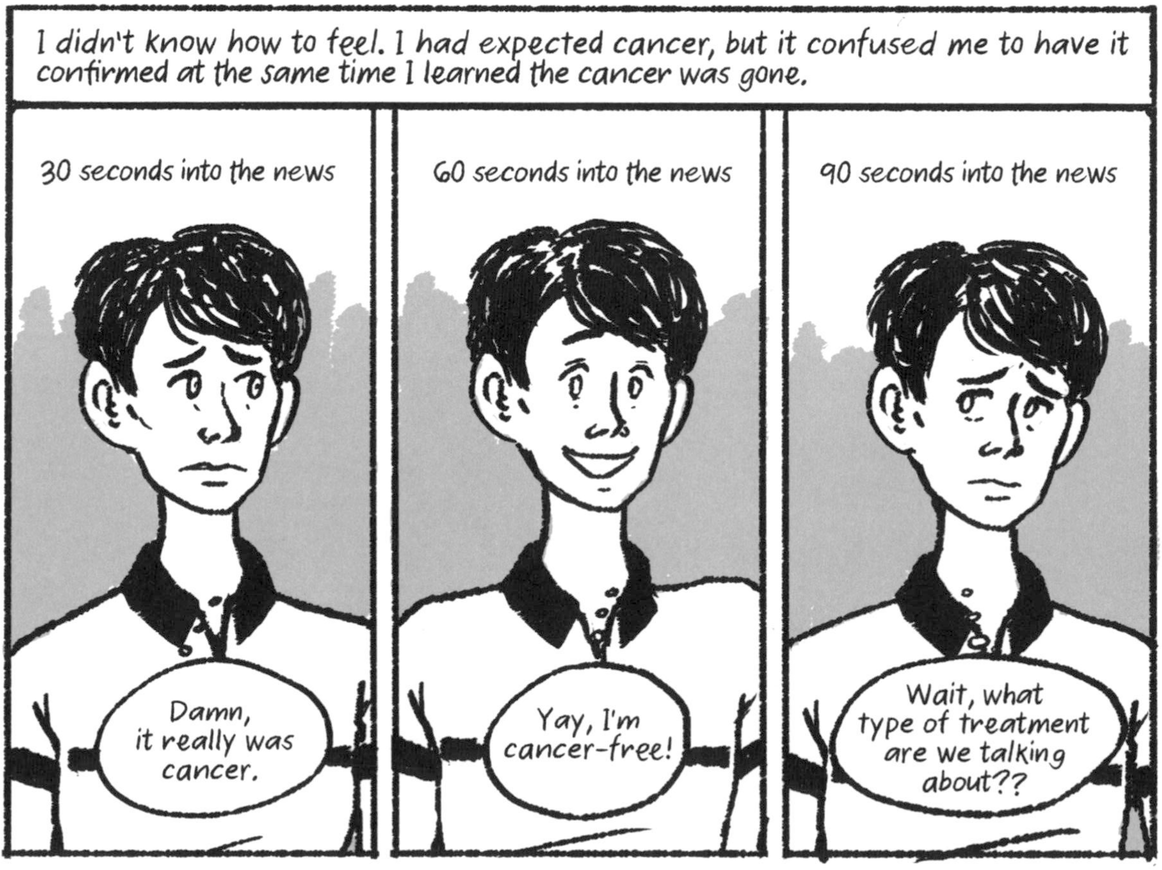
I didn't know how to feel. I had expected cancer, but it confused me to have it confirmed at the same time I learned the cancer was gone.
30 seconds into the news
Damn, it really was cancer.
60 seconds into the news
Yay, I'm cancer-free!
90 seconds into the news
Wait, what type of treatment are we talking about??

I had to make several important snap decisions about my treatment. I also had to wrestle with the fact that there was no consensus among my doctors about what caused the cancer, or even how best to proceed.

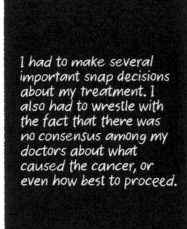

Hi Kimiko. Let's talk chemo.

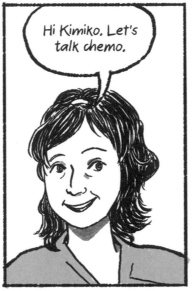

We advise sending your tumour to California to see if you need chemo. Provincial health care should cover the cost.

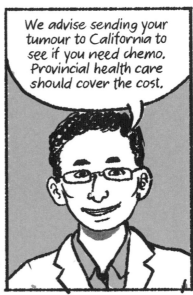

Kimiko, chemo doesn't make sense for you. We'll stick to radiation.

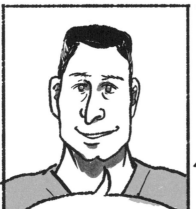

There's a risk of radiation splatter—when radiation directed at one breast spills over to the other, increasing your chance of secondary cancer.

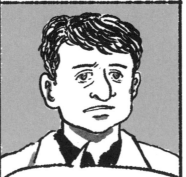

Our machines are too advanced now for radiation splatter to occur.

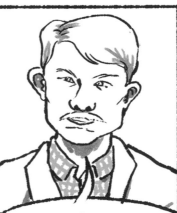

Given that your grandmother and aunt had reproductive cancers, it may be genetic.

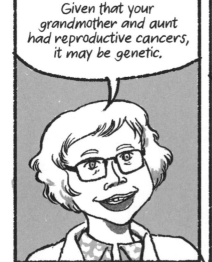

The gene test came back clear, only one variation and it may not be related. Good news is, you don't have the BRCA gene.*

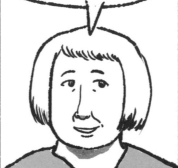

Some women consider a preventative mastectomy.

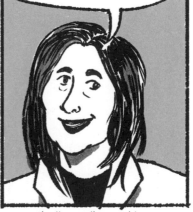

*People who have this gene are genetically predisposed to cancer.

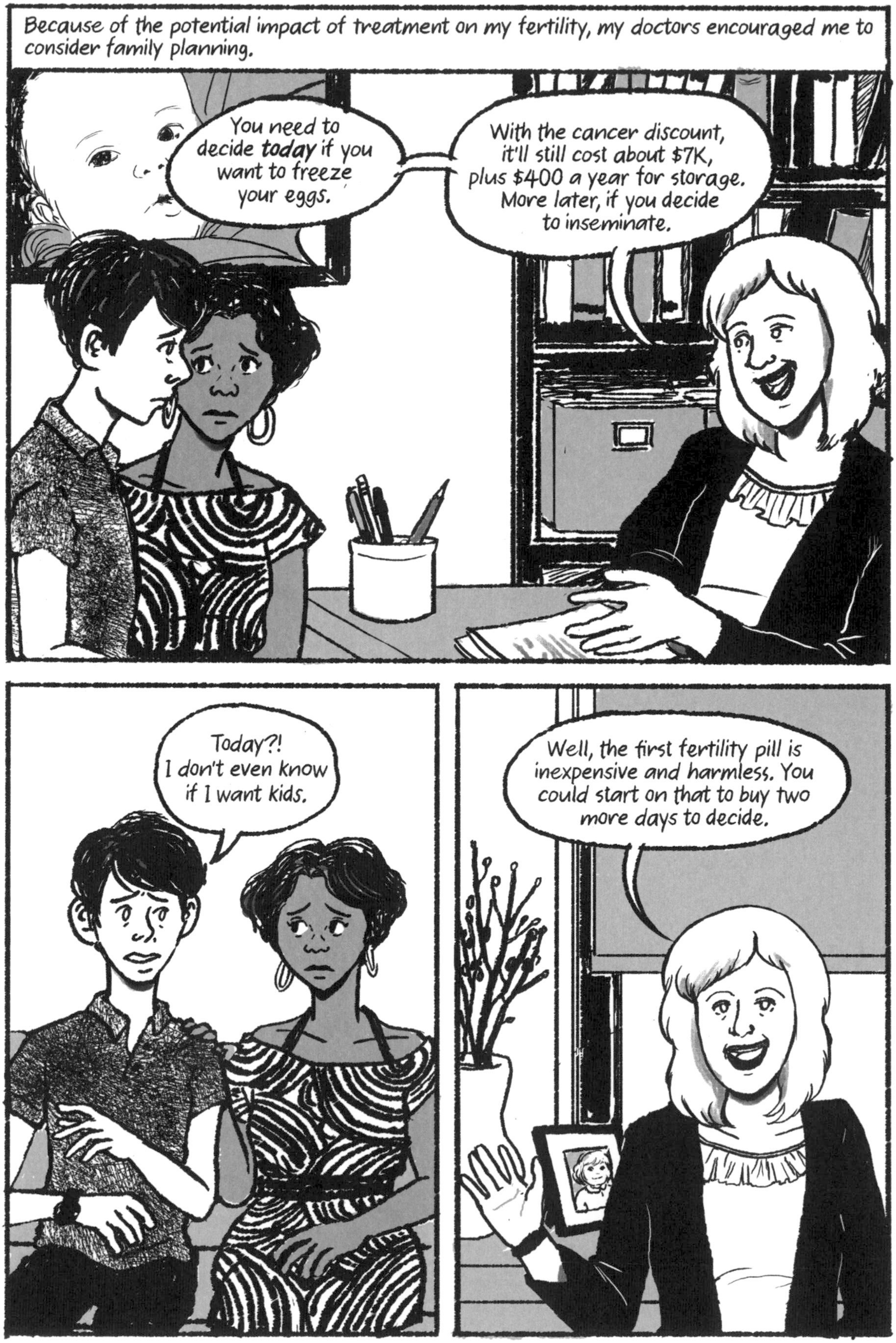
Because of the potential impact of treatment on my fertility, my doctors encouraged me to consider family planning.
You need to decide **today** if you want to freeze your eggs.
With the cancer discount, it'll still cost about $7K, plus $400 a year for storage. More later, if you decide to inseminate.
Today?! I don't even know if I want kids.
Well, the first fertility pill is inexpensive and harmless. You could start on that to buy two more days to decide.

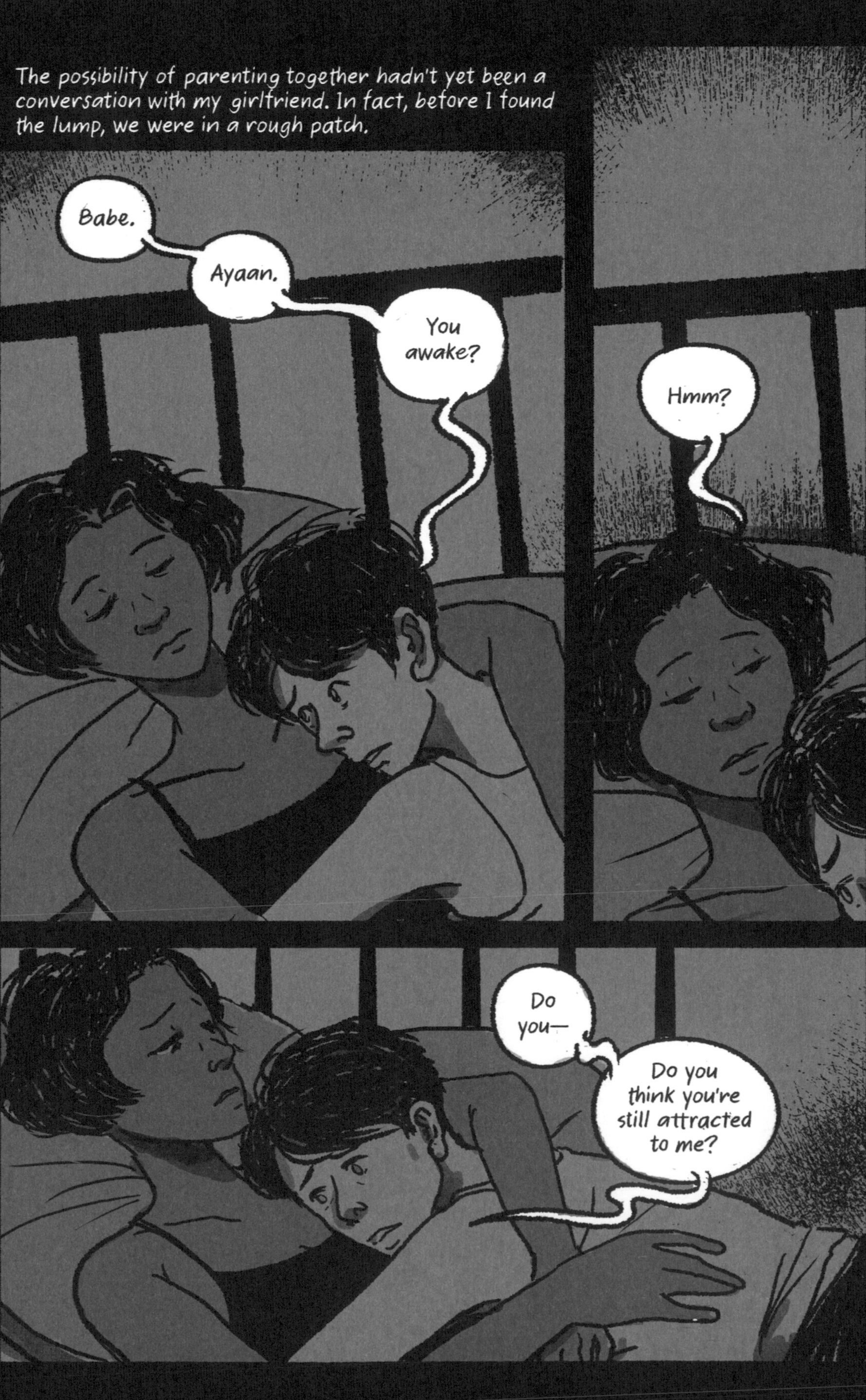
The possibility of parenting together hadn't yet been a conversation with my girlfriend. In fact, before I found the lump, we were in a rough patch.
Babe.
Ayaan.
You awake?
Hmm?
Do you—
Do you think you're still attracted to me?

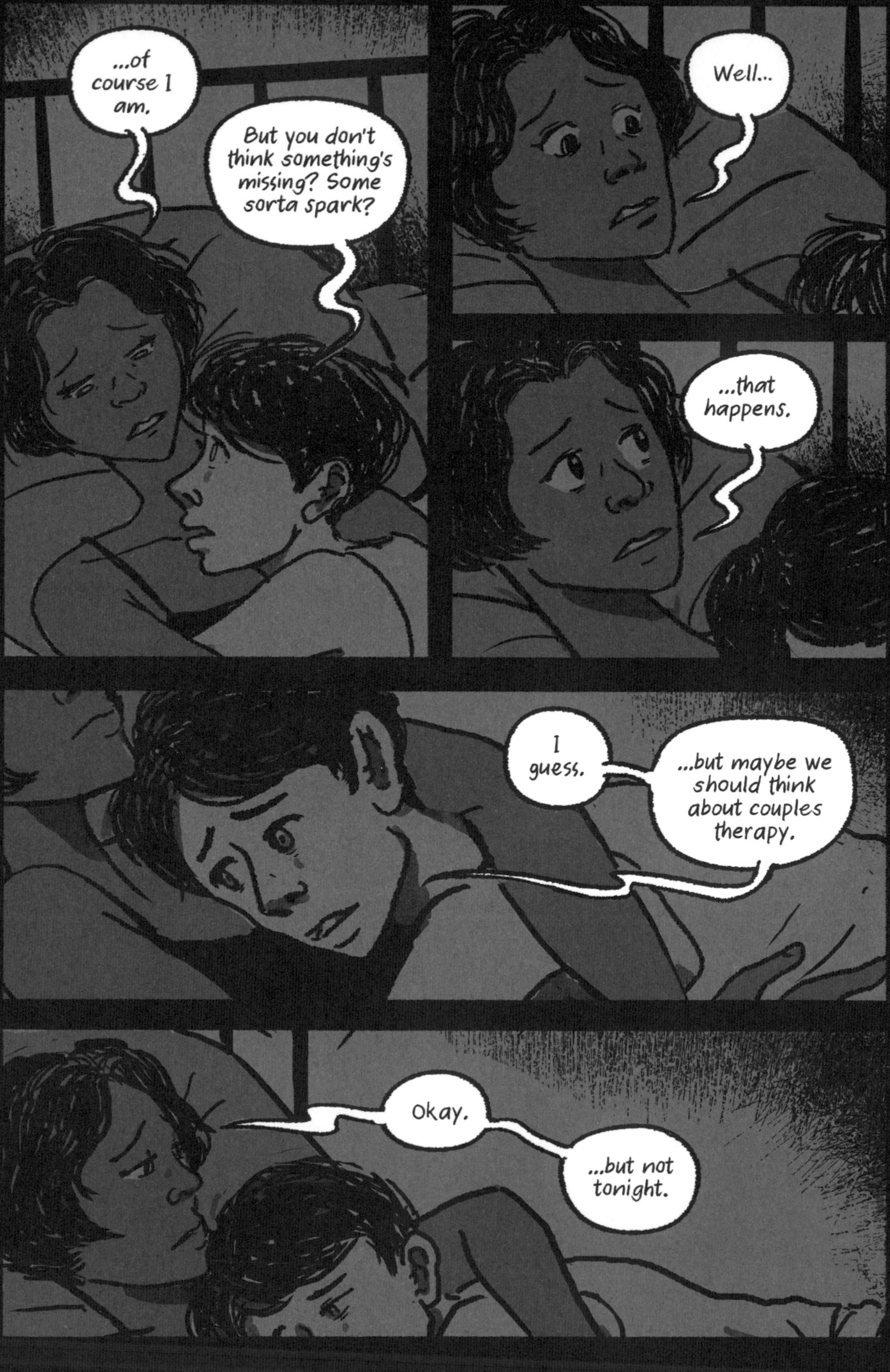
...of course I am.
But you don't think something's missing? Some sorta spark?
Well...
...that happens.
I guess.
...but maybe we should think about couples therapy.
Okay.
...but not tonight.

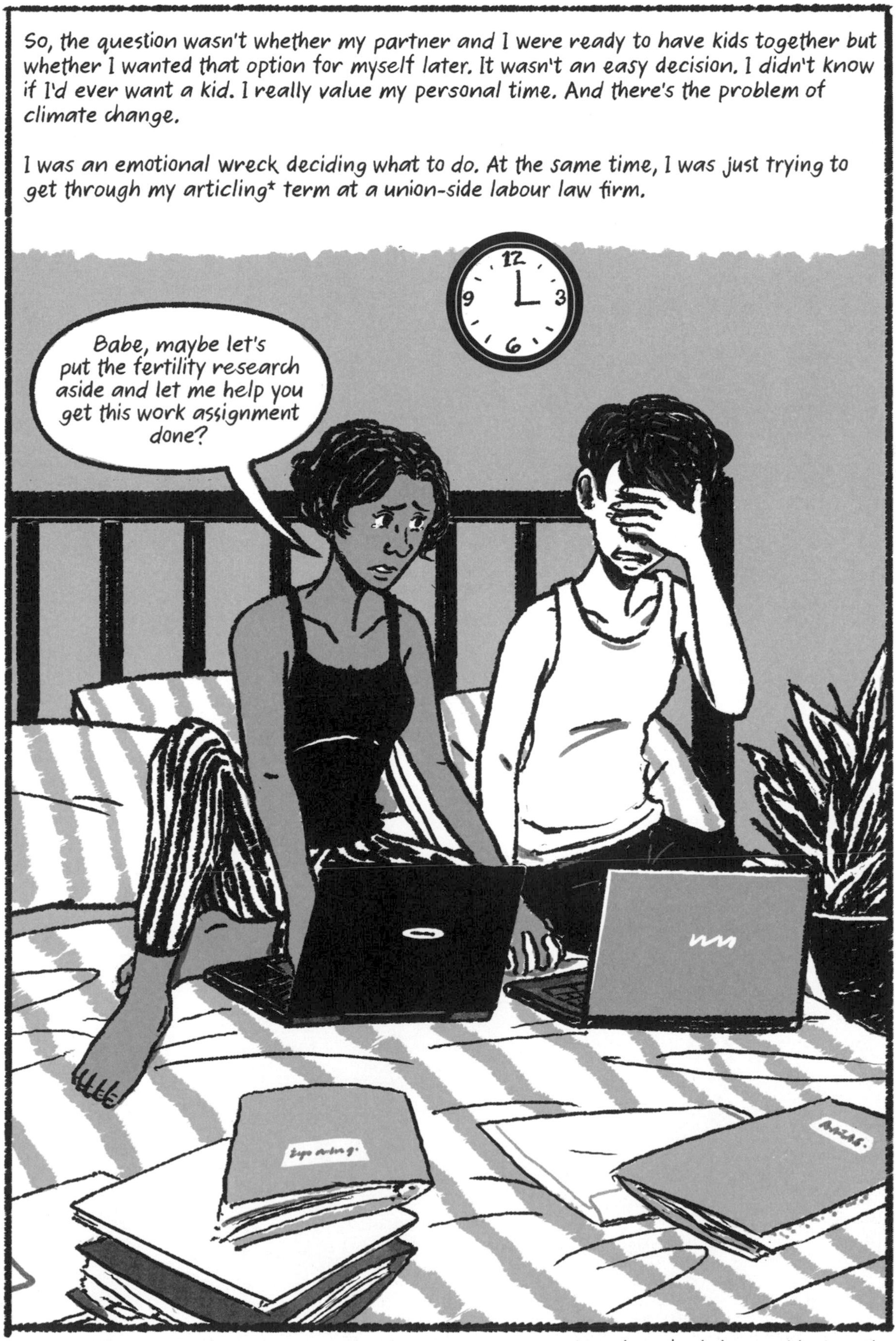
So, the question wasn't whether my partner and I were ready to have kids together but whether I wanted that option for myself later. It wasn't an easy decision. I didn't know if I'd ever want a kid. I really value my personal time. And there's the problem of climate change.
I was an emotional wreck deciding what to do. At the same time, I was just trying to get through my articling* term at a union-side labour law firm.
Babe, maybe let's put the fertility research aside and let me help you get this work assignment done?

*Post-law school placement in Canada.

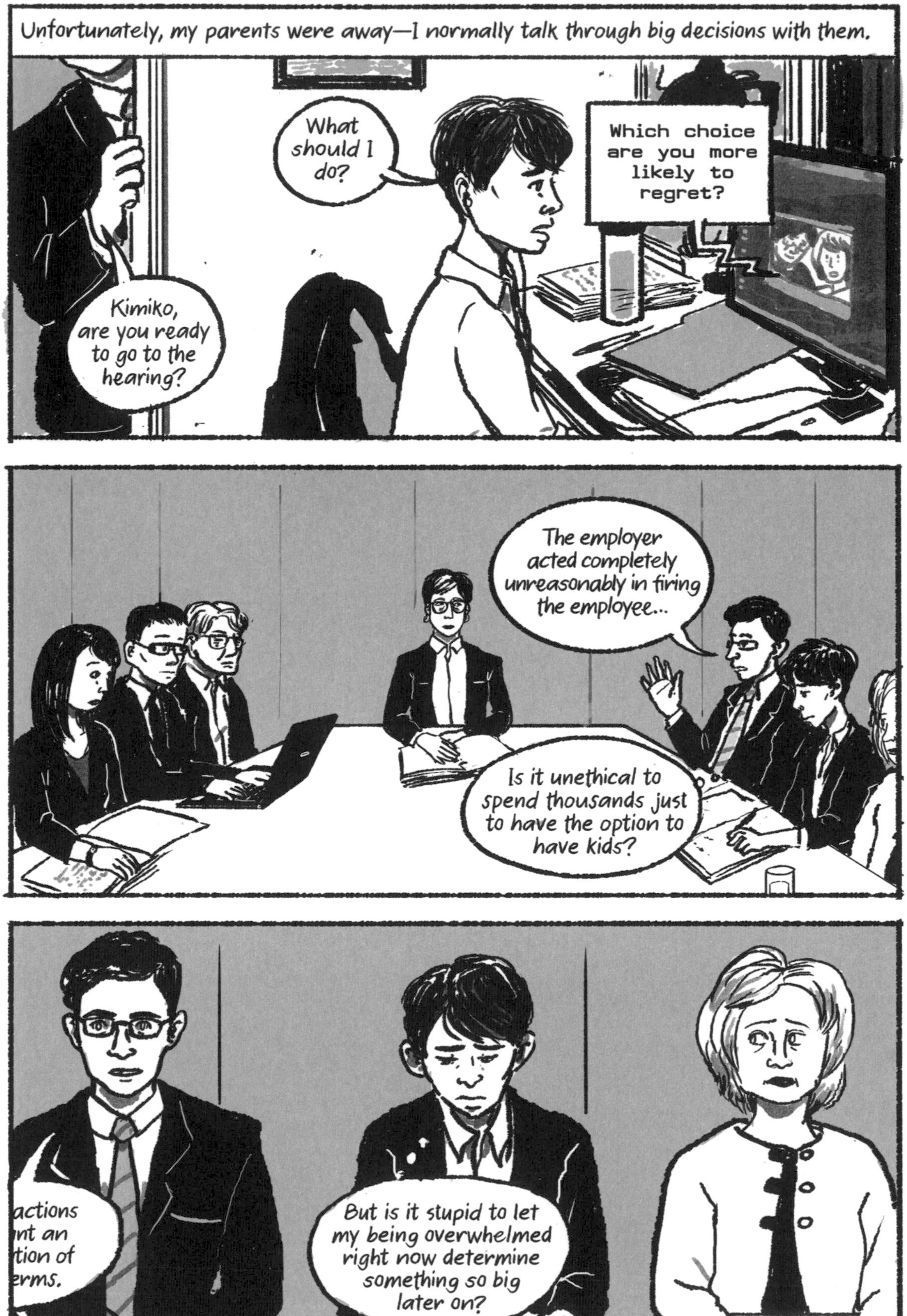
Unfortunately, my parents were away—I normally talk through big decisions with them.
Kimiko, are you ready to go to the hearing?
What should I do?
Which choice are you more likely to regret?
The employer acted completely unreasonably in firing the employee...
Is it unethical to spend thousands just to have the option to have kids?
actions
nt an
tion of
erms.
But is it stupid to let my being overwhelmed right now determine something so big later on?

In the end, I told myself that Future Me would forgive Present Me for whatever I decided. So, because I could afford it, I went with what left me the most options.

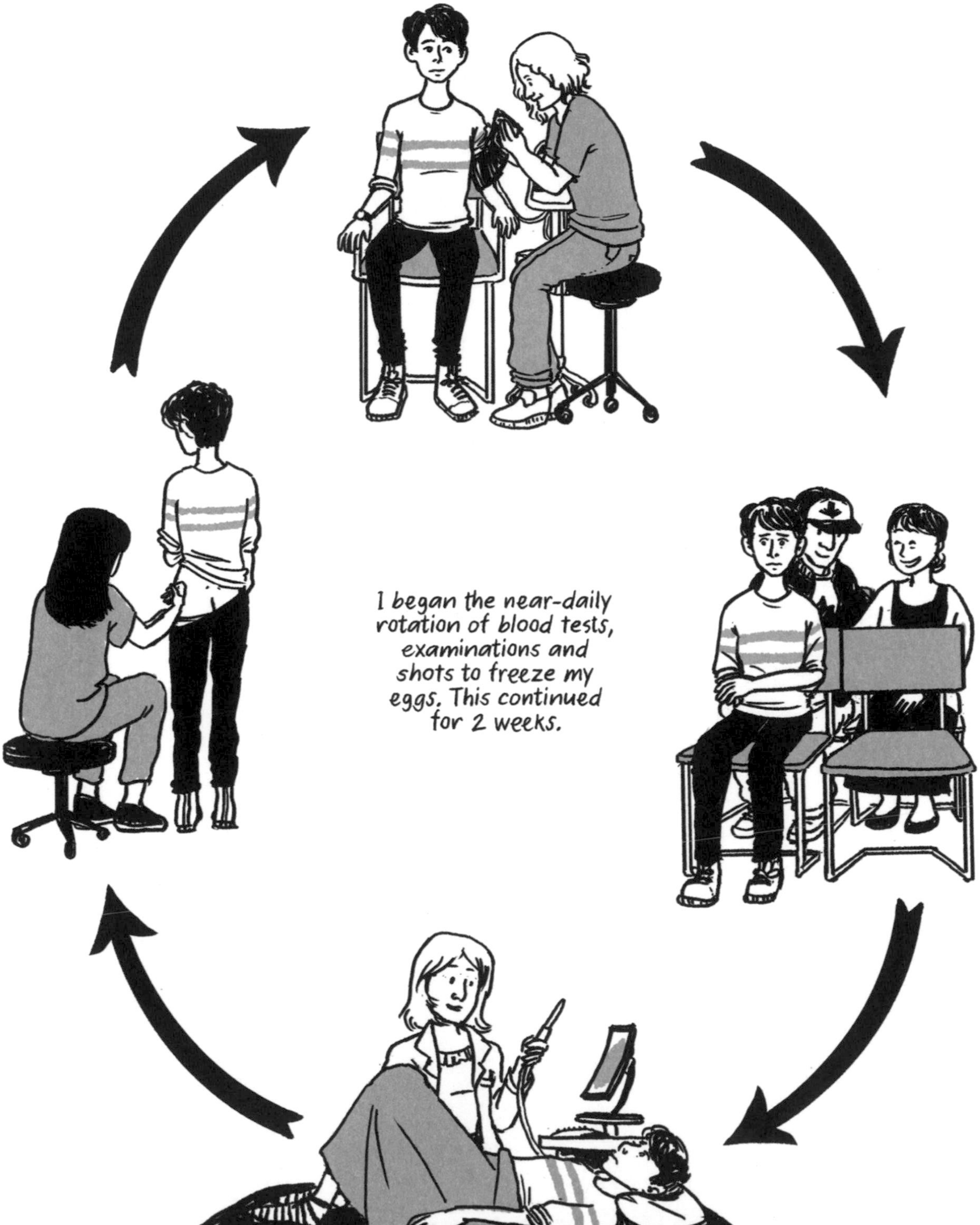
I began the near-daily rotation of blood tests, examinations and shots to freeze my eggs. This continued for 2 weeks.

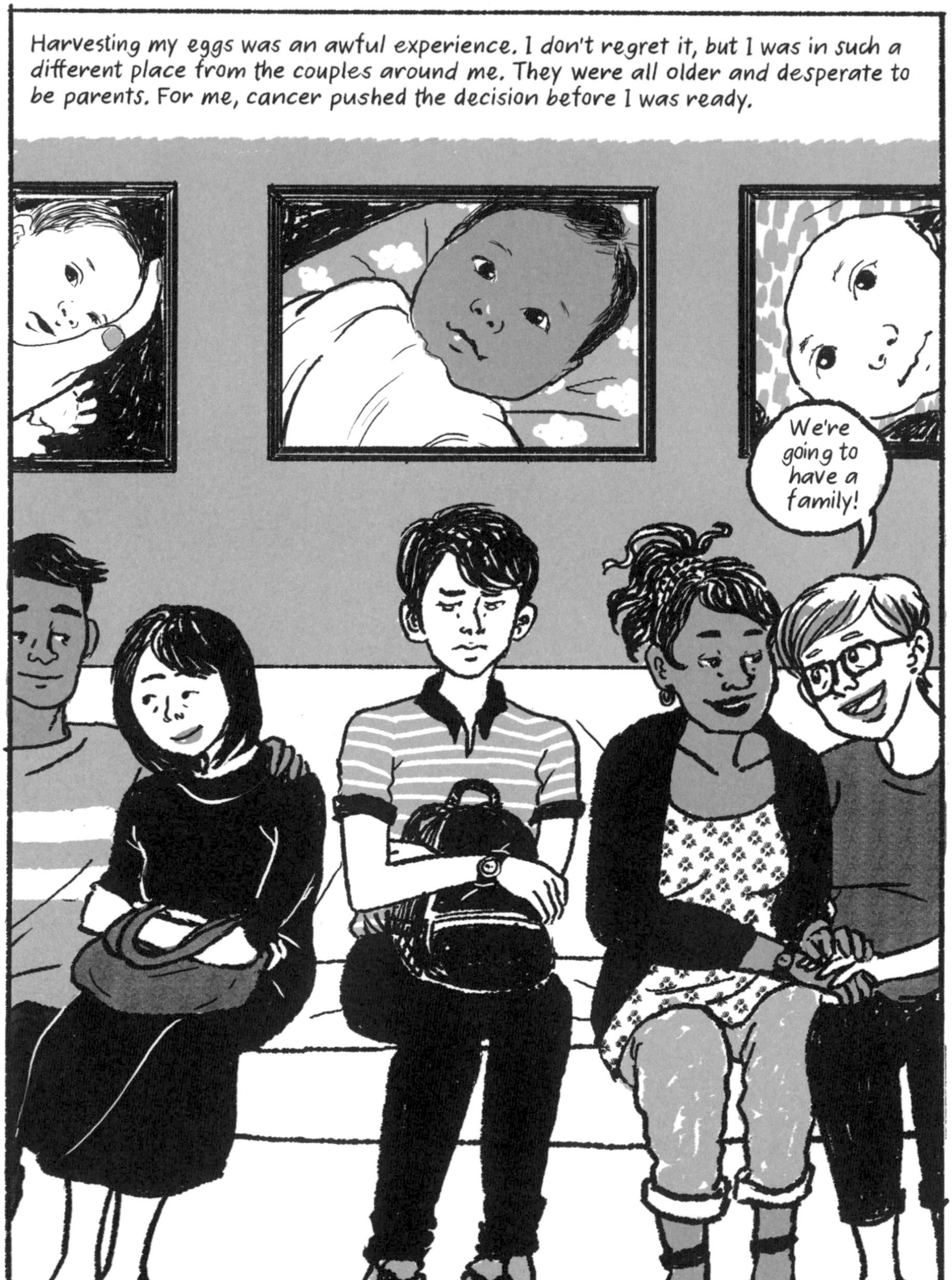
Harvesting my eggs was an awful experience. I don't regret it, but I was in such a different place from the couples around me. They were all older and desperate to be parents. For me, cancer pushed the decision before I was ready.
We're going to have a family!
In case you're wondering, they harvested 28 eggs. That's a lot of eggs on the rocks. I'm considering starting a side business if the whole lawyer thing doesn't pan out...

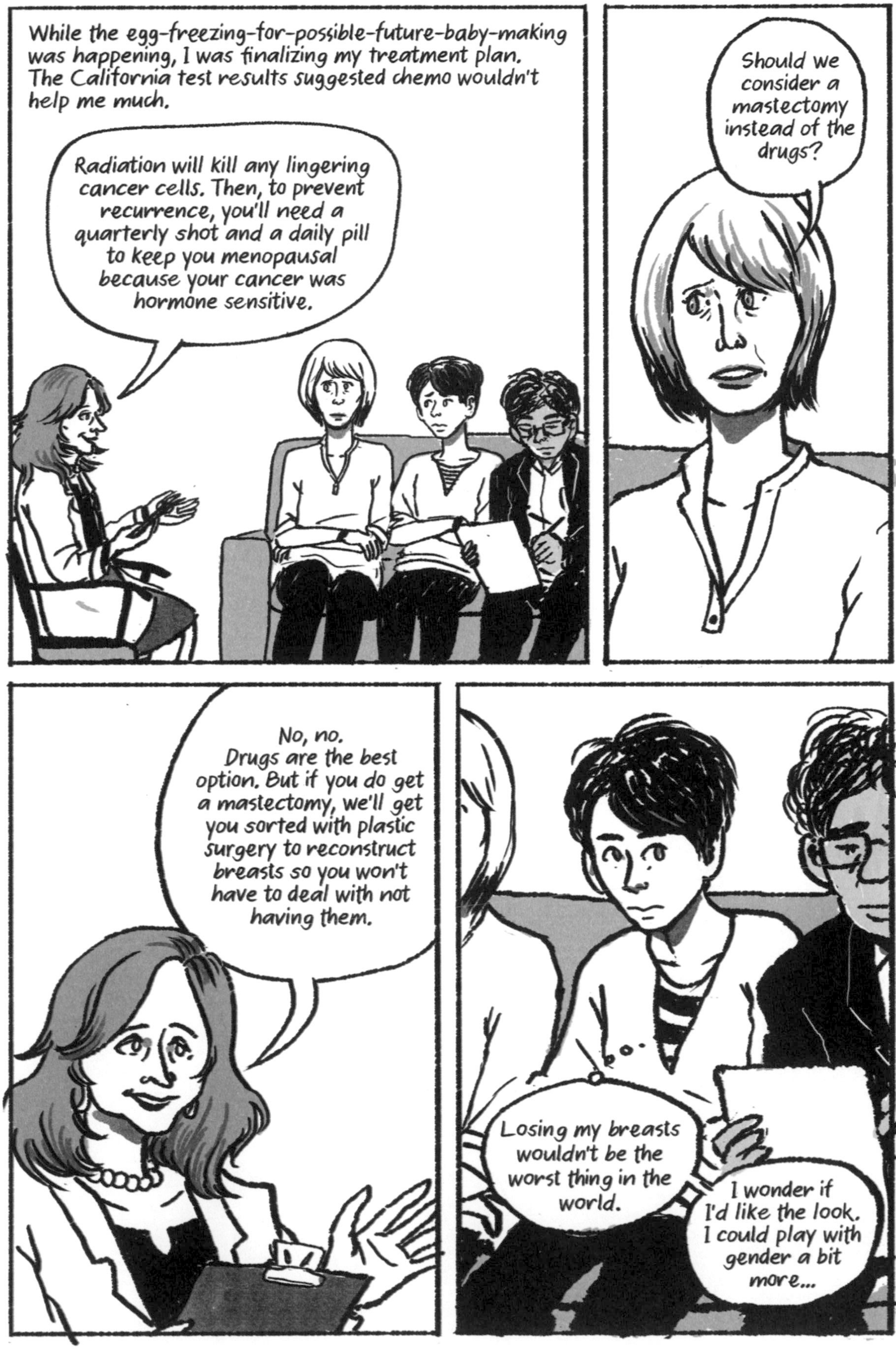
While the egg-freezing-for-possible-future-baby-making was happening, I was finalizing my treatment plan. The California test results suggested chemo wouldn't help me much.
Radiation will kill any lingering cancer cells. Then, to prevent recurrence, you'll need a quarterly shot and a daily pill to keep you menopausal because your cancer was hormone sensitive.
Should we consider a mastectomy instead of the drugs?
No, no. Drugs are the best option. But if you do get a mastectomy, we'll get you sorted with plastic surgery to reconstruct breasts so you won't have to deal with not having them.
Losing my breasts wouldn't be the worst thing in the world.
I wonder if I'd like the look. I could play with gender a bit more...

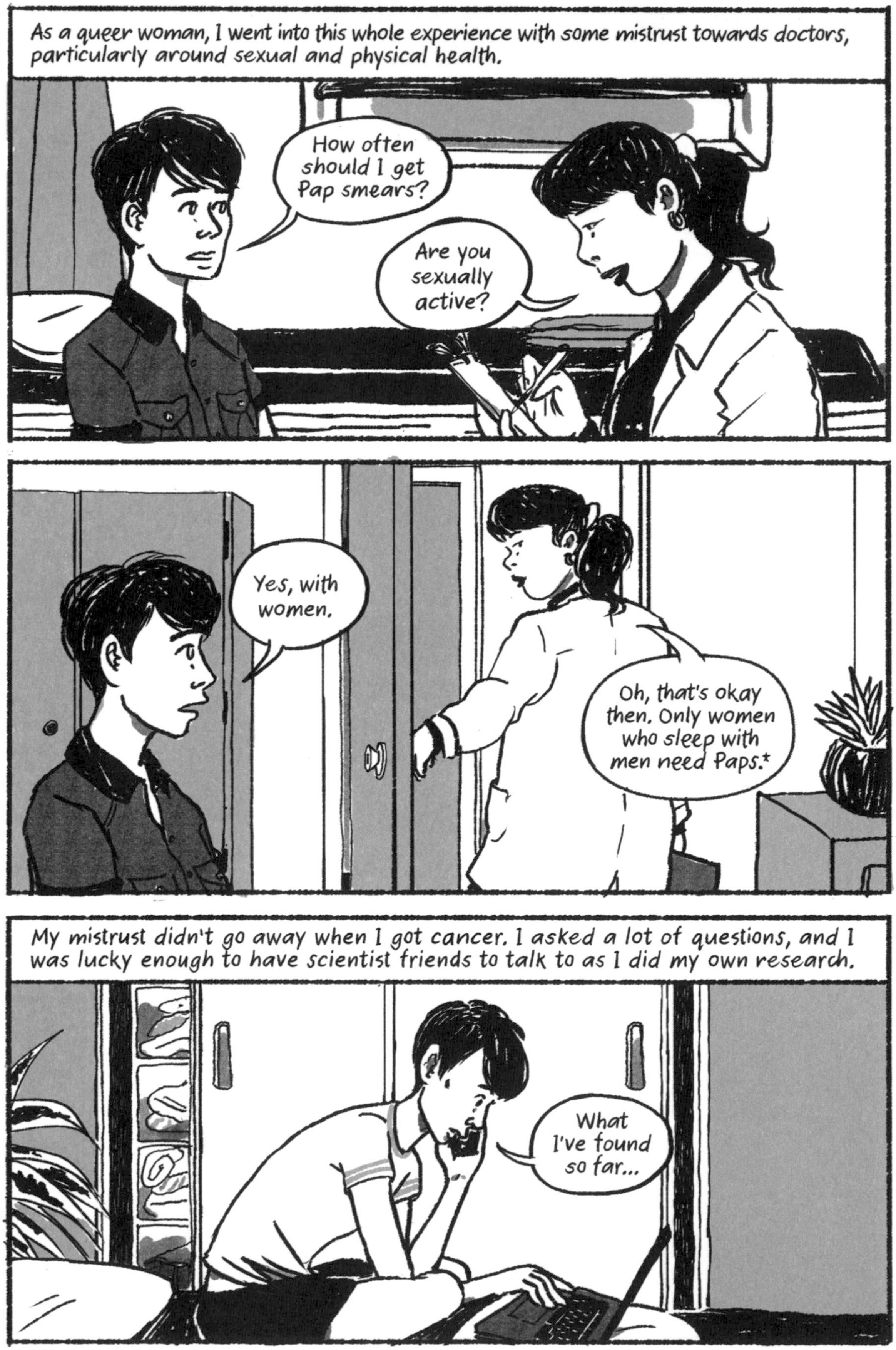
As a queer woman, I went into this whole experience with some mistrust towards doctors, particularly around sexual and physical health.
How often should I get Pap smears?
Are you sexually active?
Yes, with women.
Oh, that's okay then. Only women who sleep with men need Paps.*
My mistrust didn't go away when I got cancer. I asked a lot of questions, and I was lucky enough to have scientist friends to talk to as I did my own research.
What I've found so far...

*Bad medical advice.

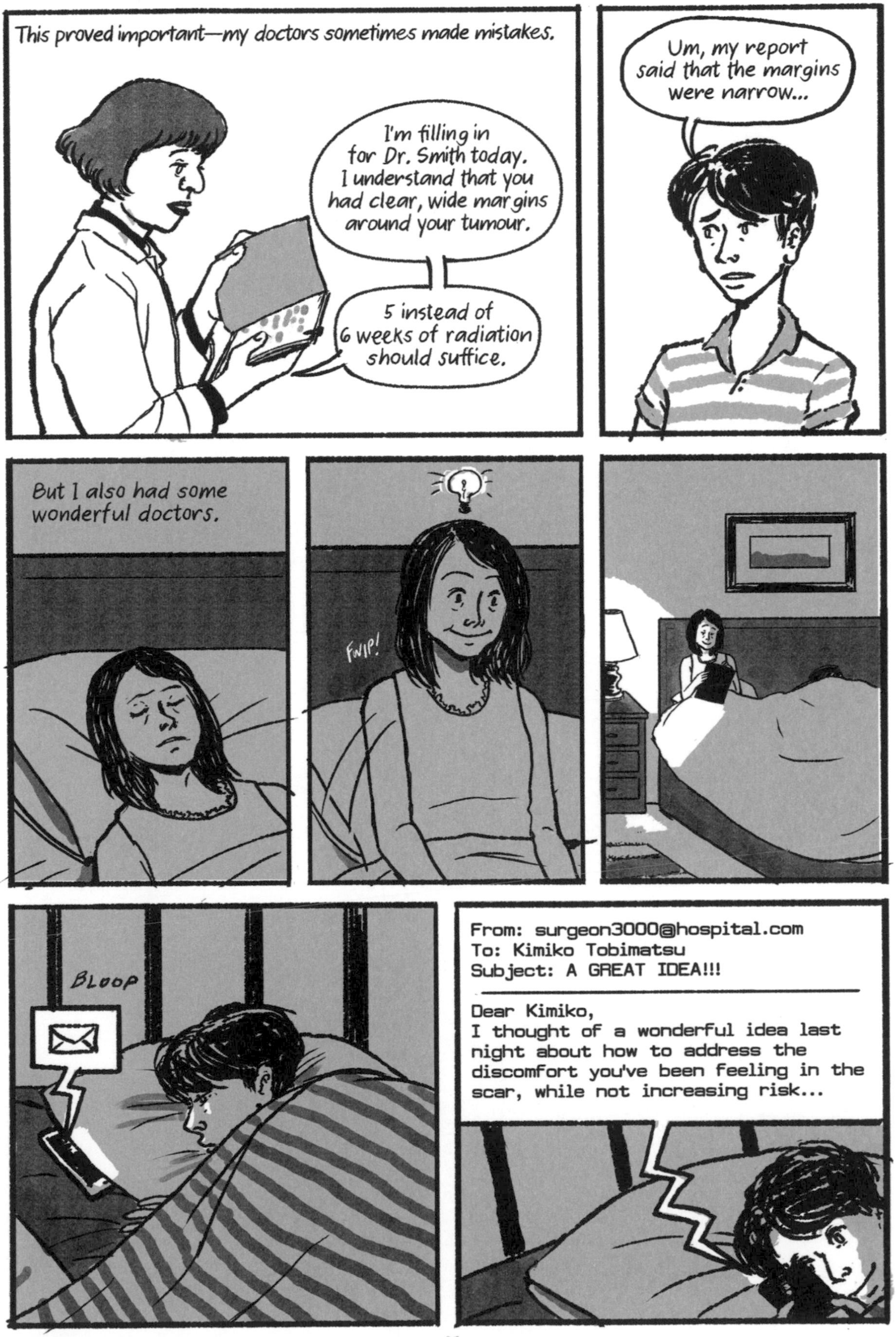
This proved important—my doctors sometimes made mistakes.
I'm filling in for Dr. Smith today. I understand that you had clear, wide margins around your tumour.
5 instead of 6 weeks of radiation should suffice.
Um, my report said that the margins were narrow...
But I also had some wonderful doctors.
FWIP!
BLOOP
From: surgeon3000@hospital.com
To: Kimiko Tobimatsu
Subject: A GREAT IDEA!!!
Dear Kimiko,
I thought of a wonderful idea last night about how to address the discomfort you've been feeling in the scar, while not increasing risk...

In no time at all, I had more medical practitioners than my 95-year-old obaachan.

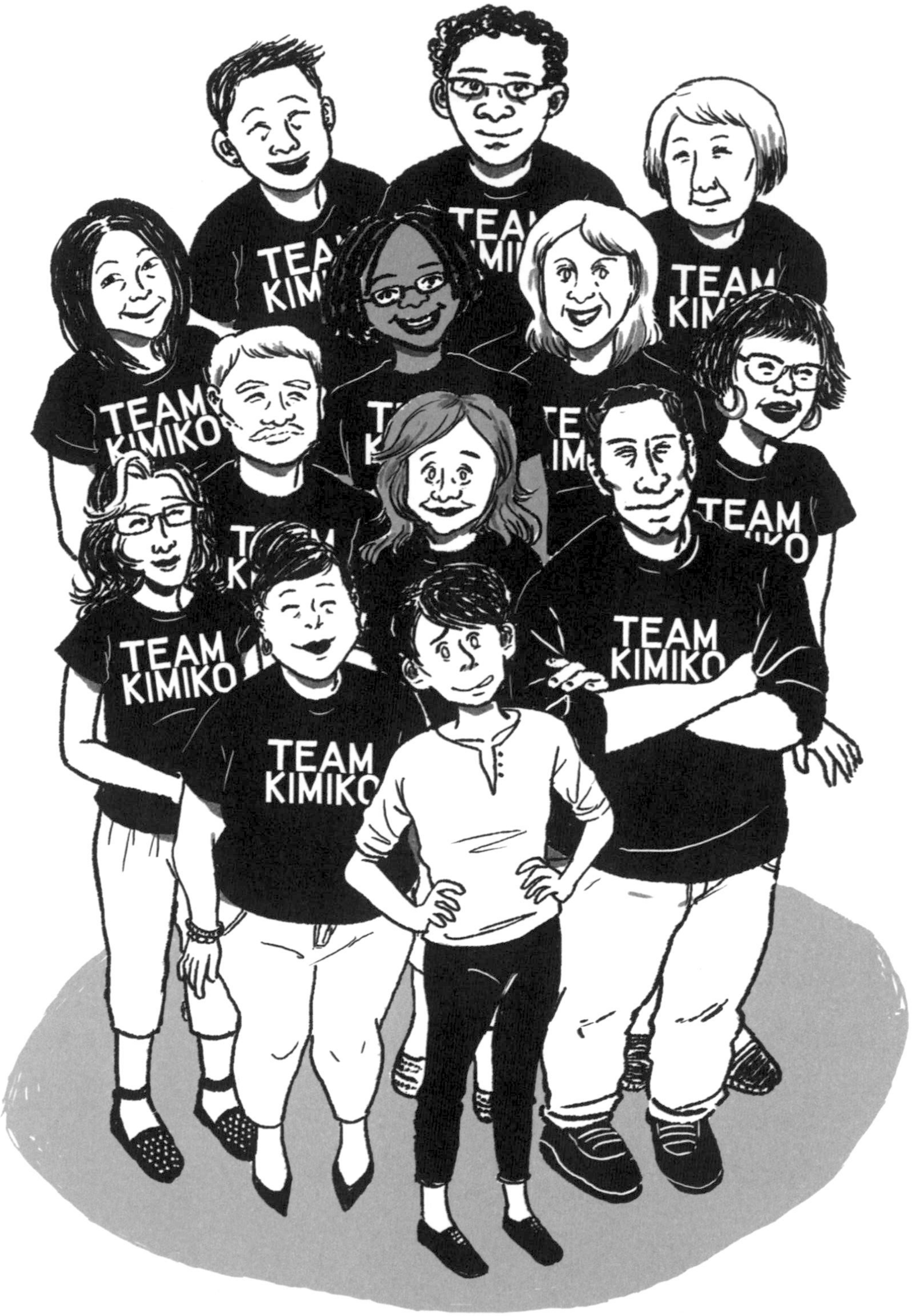
TEAM
KIMIKO

Now I understand why people talk about having a medical "team." I'd thought it was just one of those culty cancer things, like nurses being called angels, but I realized that it merely reflects the sheer number of health care workers assigned to each patient. Which, while amazing,* also had me feeling that I was being tossed from person to person and had little agency (and I say that as someone with a much greater capacity to advocate for myself than the average patient).

*Especially so given Canada's universal health care system.

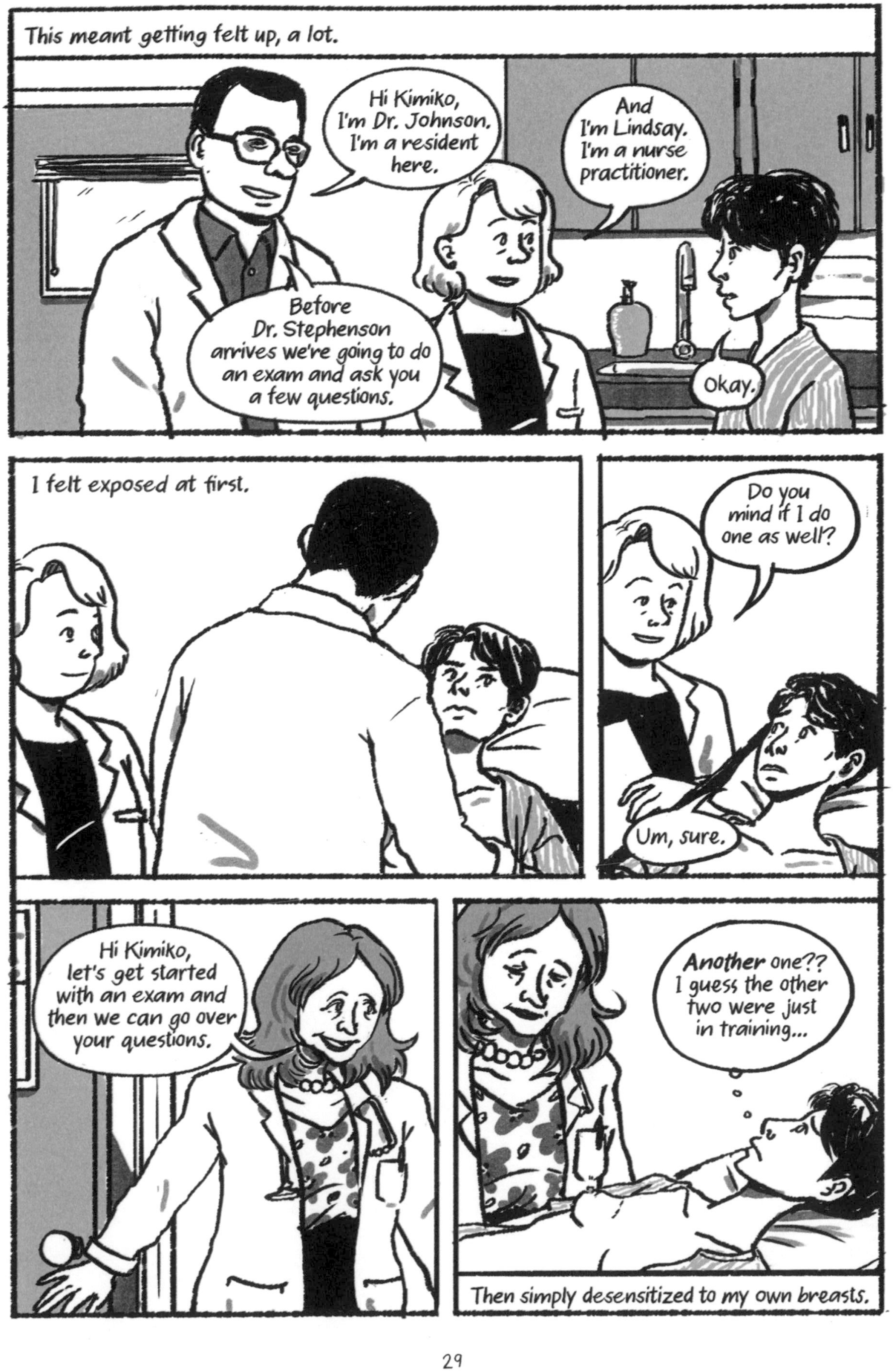
This meant getting felt up, a lot.
Hi Kimiko, I'm Dr. Johnson. I'm a resident here.
And I'm Lindsay. I'm a nurse practitioner.
Before Dr. Stephenson arrives we're going to do an exam and ask you a few questions.
Okay.
I felt exposed at first.
Do you mind if I do one as well?
Um, sure.
Hi Kimiko, let's get started with an exam and then we can go over your questions.
Another one?? I guess the other two were just in training...
Then simply desensitized to my own breasts.

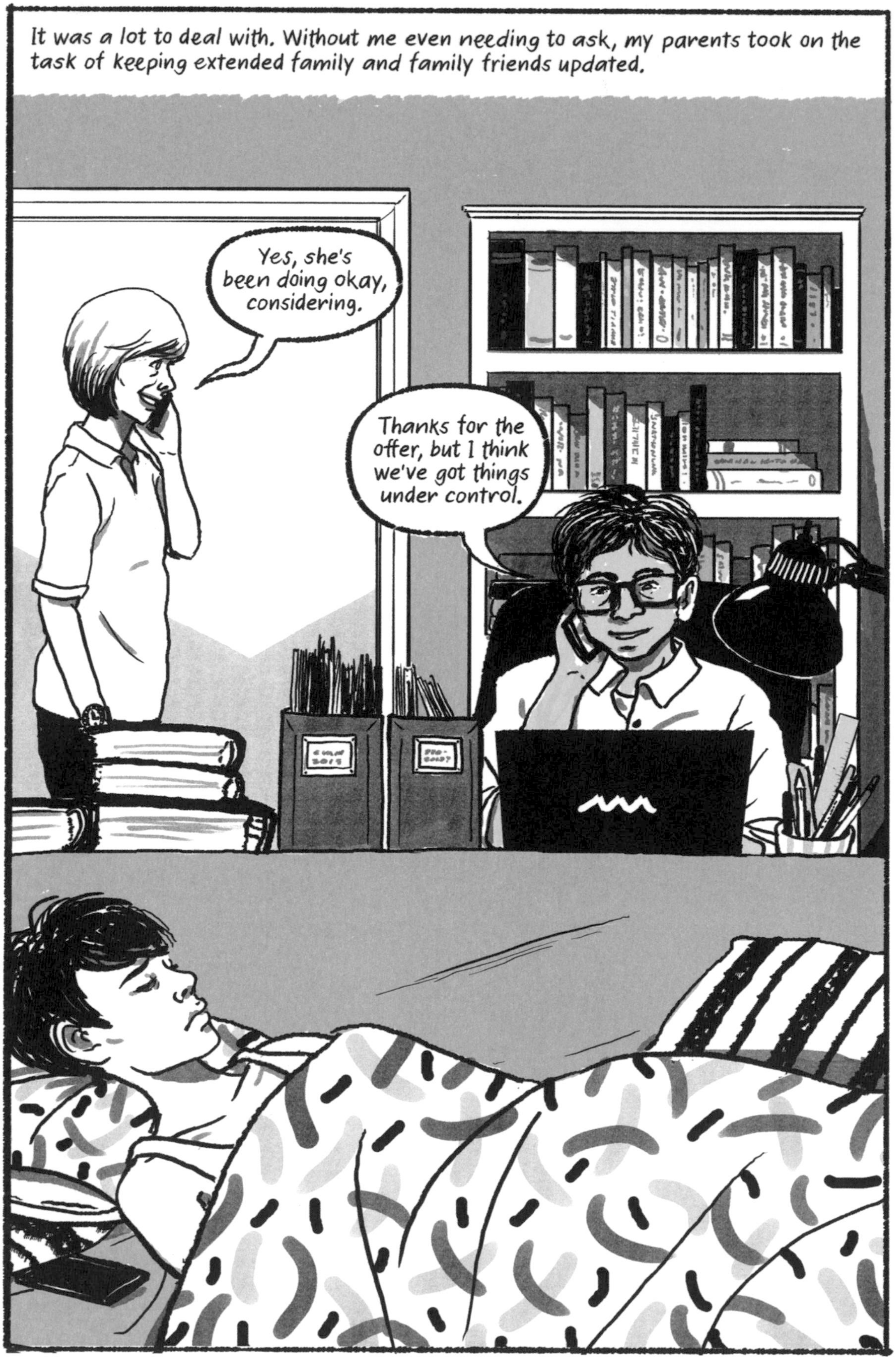
It was a lot to deal with. Without me even needing to ask, my parents took on the task of keeping extended family and family friends updated.
Yes, she's been doing okay, considering.
Thanks for the offer, but I think we've got things under control.

My partner also played a huge part in getting me through that first year. Our relationship concerns were still there, but, for better or worse, they took the back seat.

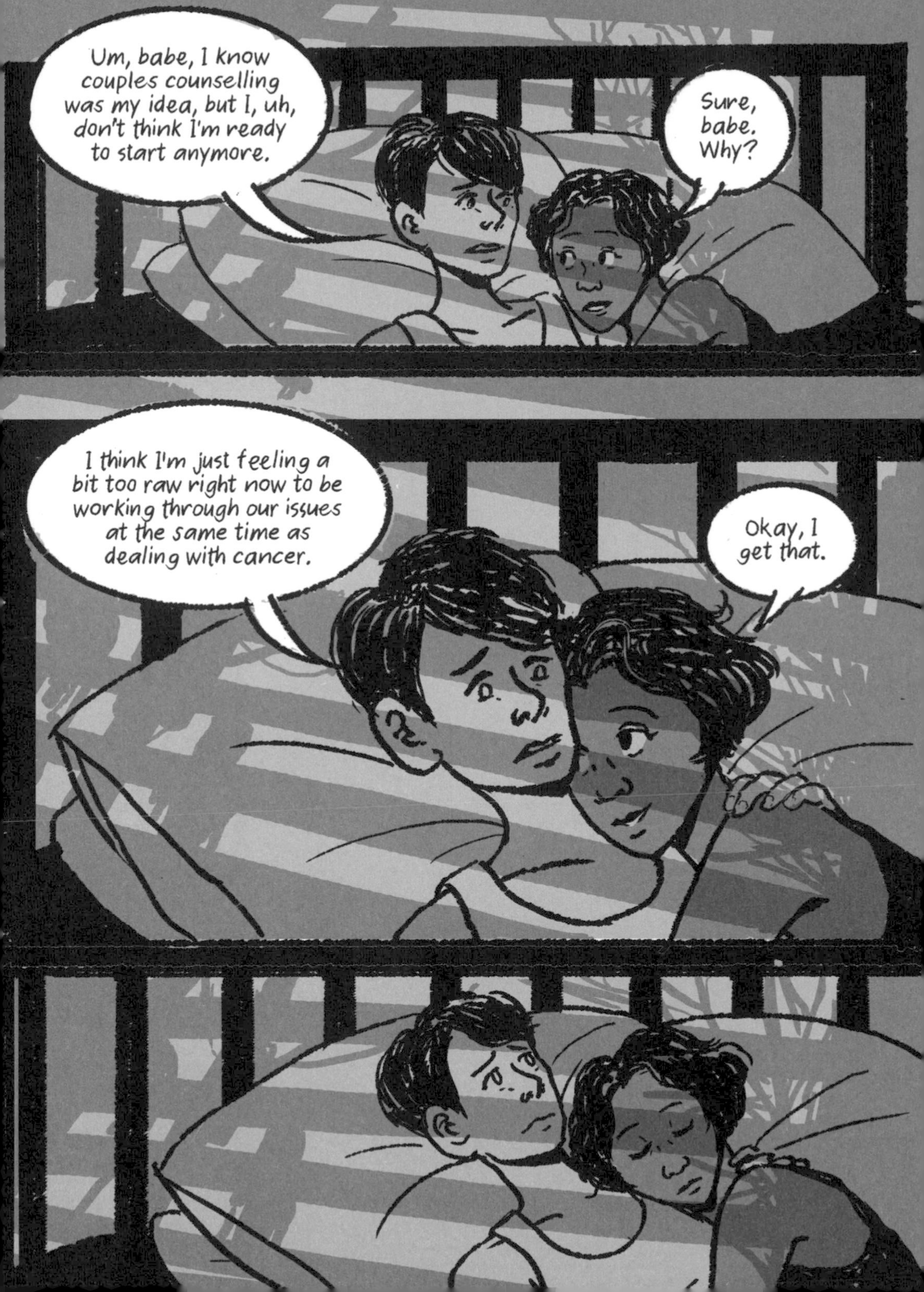
Um, babe, I know couples counselling was my idea, but I, uh, don't think I'm ready to start anymore.
Sure, babe. Why?
I think I'm just feeling a bit too raw right now to be working through our issues at the same time as dealing with cancer.
Okay, I get that.

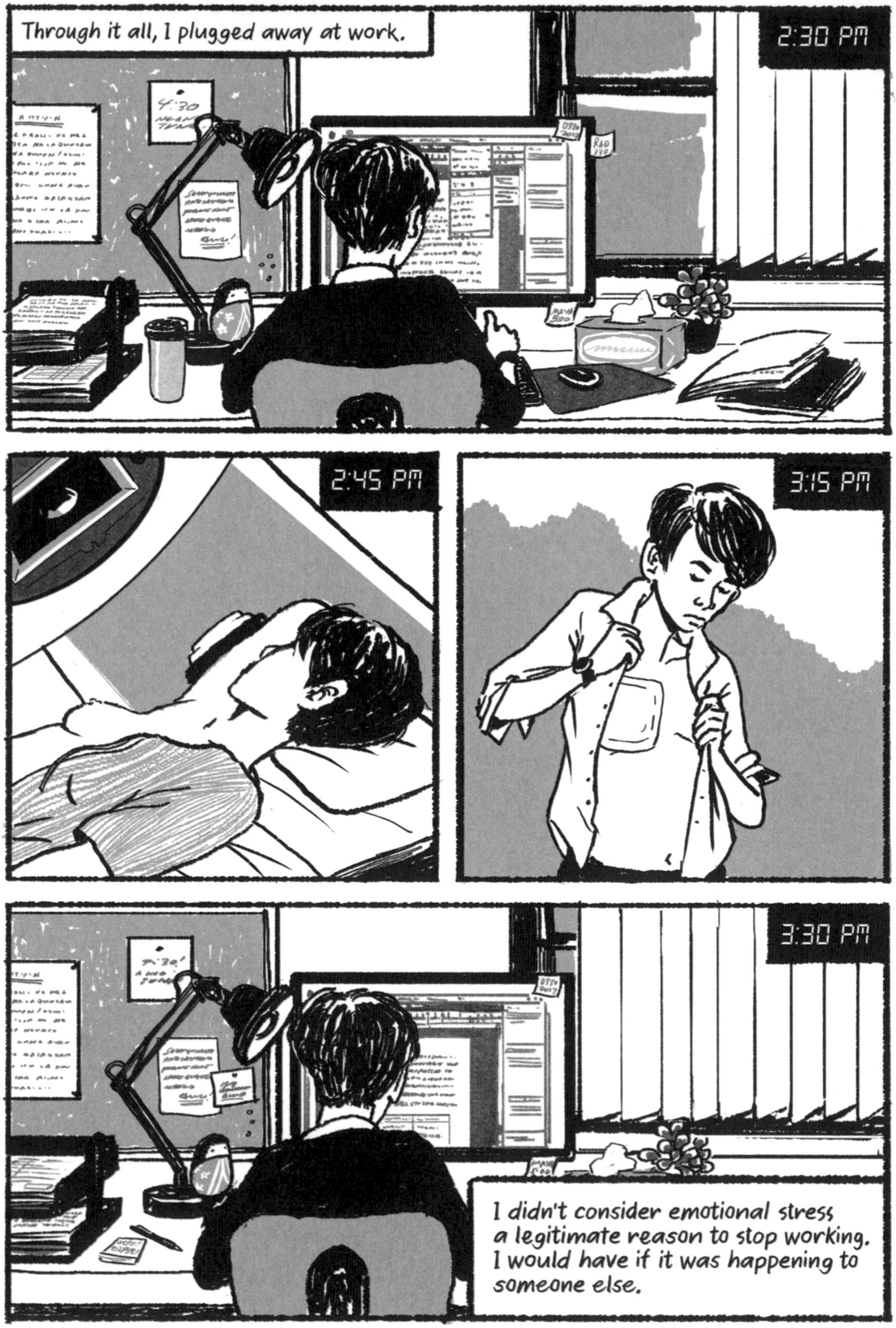
Through it all, I plugged away at work.
2:30 PM
2:45 PM
3:15 PM
3:30 PM
I didn't consider emotional stress a legitimate reason to stop working. I would have if it was happening to someone else.

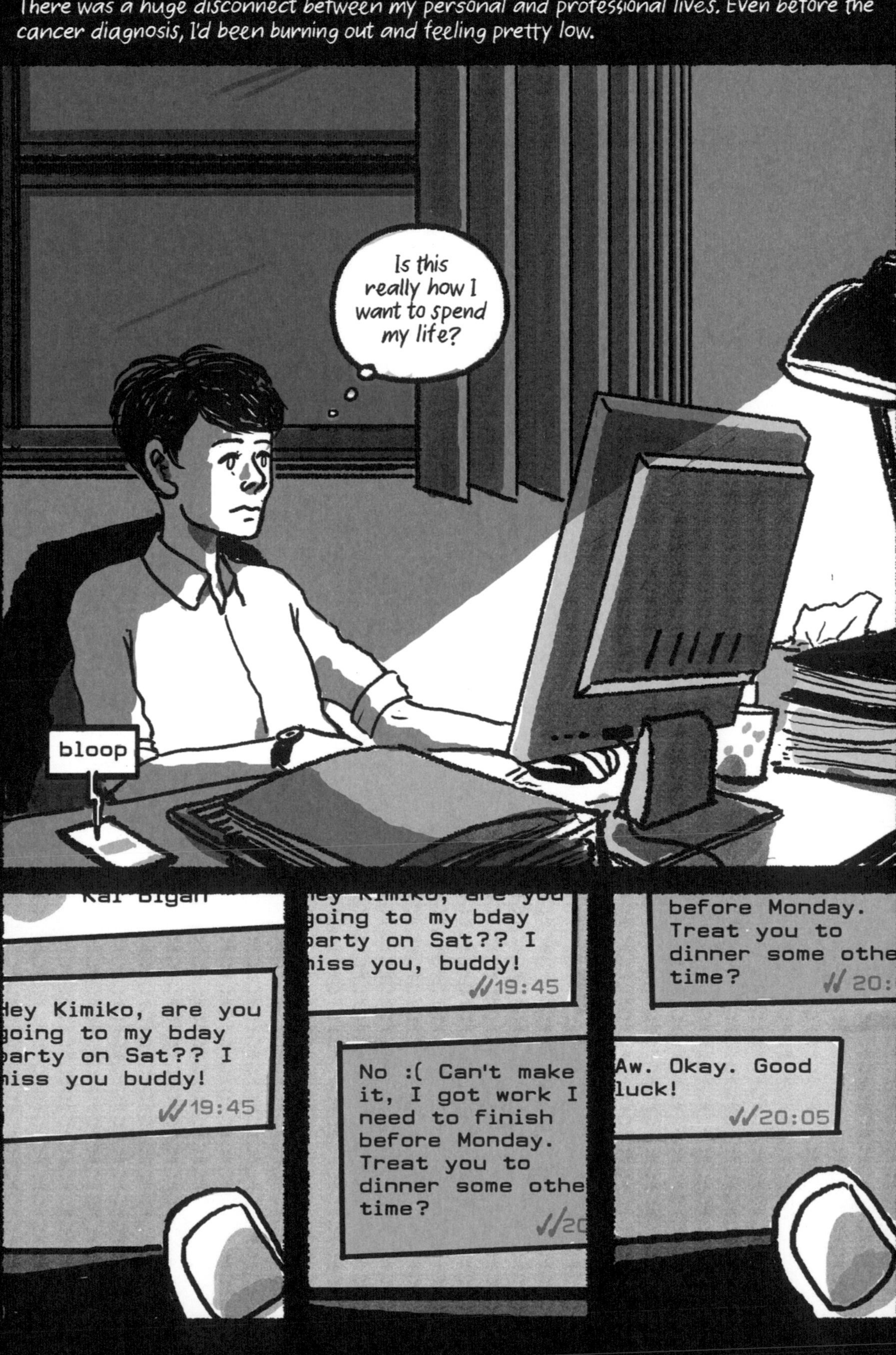

There was a huge disconnect between my personal and professional lives. Even before the cancer diagnosis, I'd been burning out and feeling pretty low.
Is this really how I want to spend my life?
bloop
ey Kimiko, are you oing to my bday arty on Sat?? I iss you buddy!
19:45
oing to my bday arty on Sat?? I iss you, buddy!
19:45
No :(Can't make it, I got work I need to finish before Monday. Treat you to dinner some othe time?
before Monday. Treat you to dinner some othe time?
Aw. Okay. Good luck!
20:05

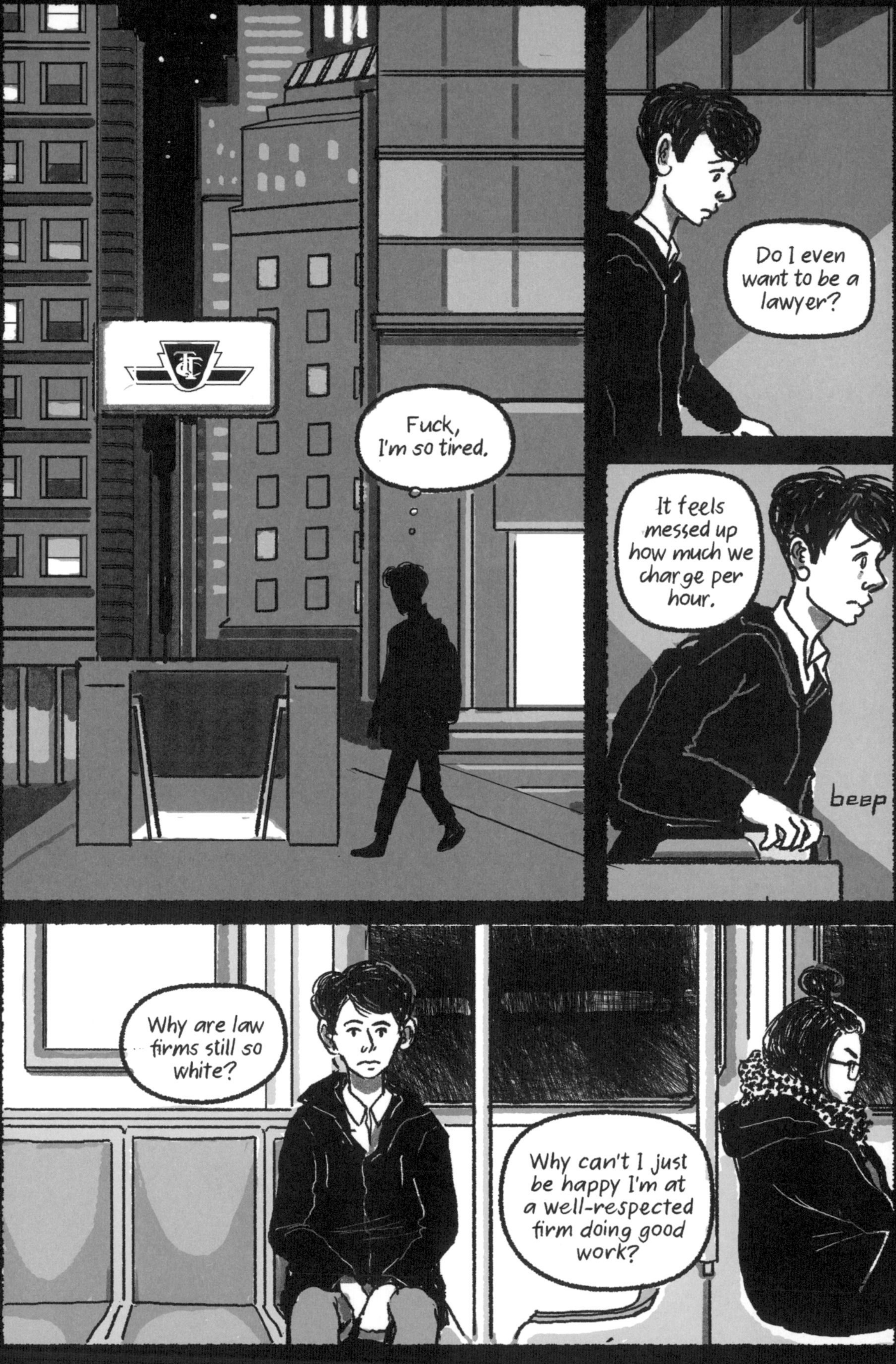
Fuck, I'm so tired.
Do I even want to be a lawyer?
It feels messed up how much we charge per hour.
beep
Why are law firms still so white?
Why can't I just be happy I'm at a well-respected firm doing good work?

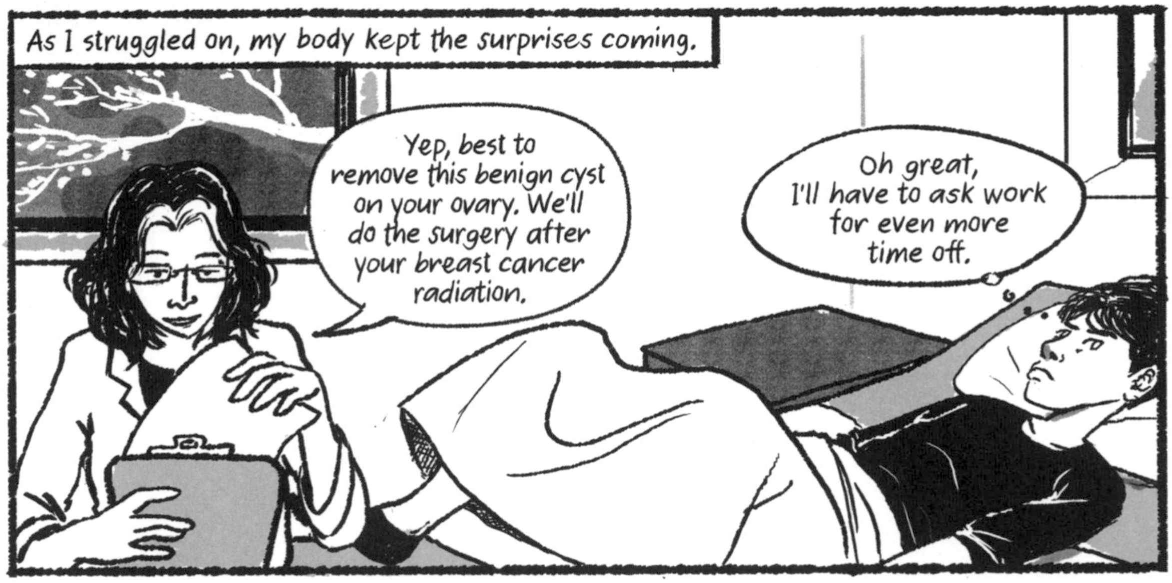
As I struggled on, my body kept the surprises coming.
Yep, best to remove this benign cyst on your ovary. We'll do the surgery after your breast cancer radiation.
Oh great, I'll have to ask work for even more time off.

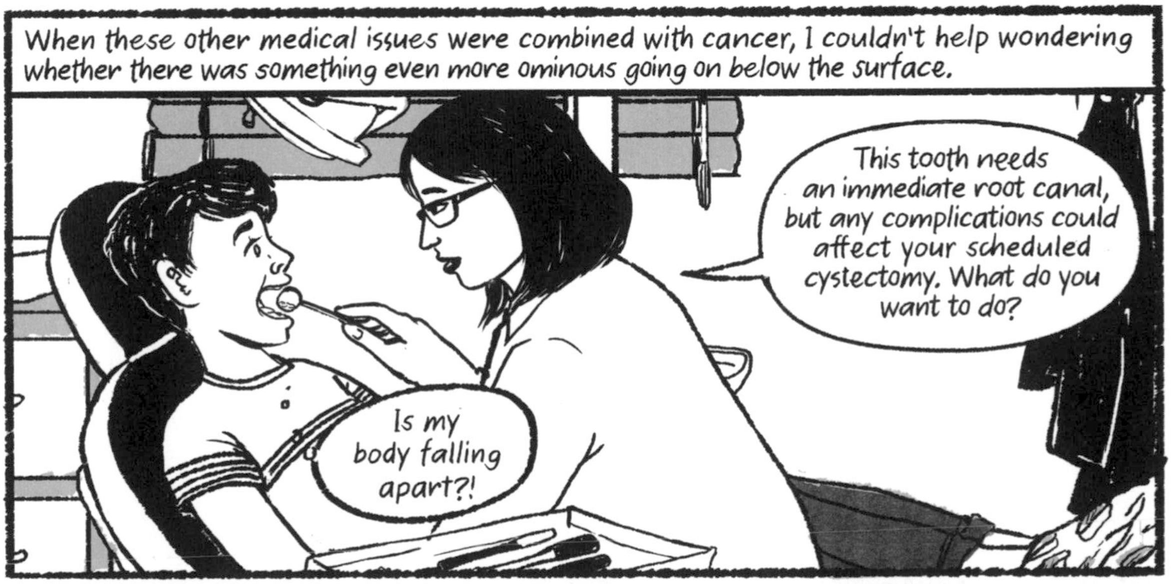
When these other medical issues were combined with cancer, I couldn't help wondering whether there was something even more ominous going on below the surface.
This tooth needs an immediate root canal, but any complications could affect your scheduled cystectomy. What do you want to do?
Is my body falling apart?!

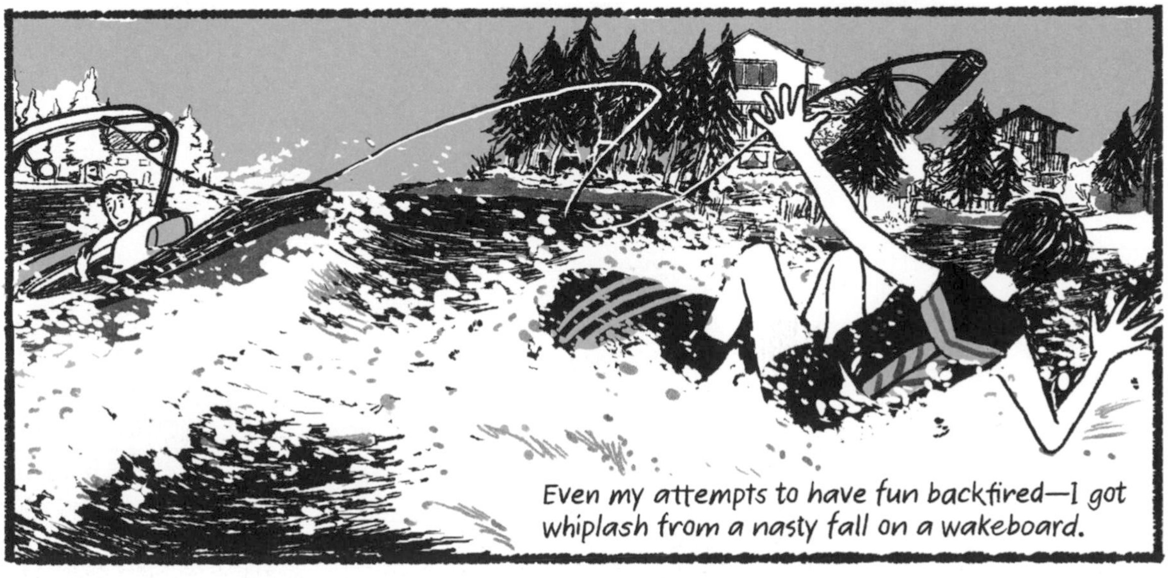
Even my attempts to have fun backfired—I got whiplash from a nasty fall on a wakeboard.

THE OTHERS

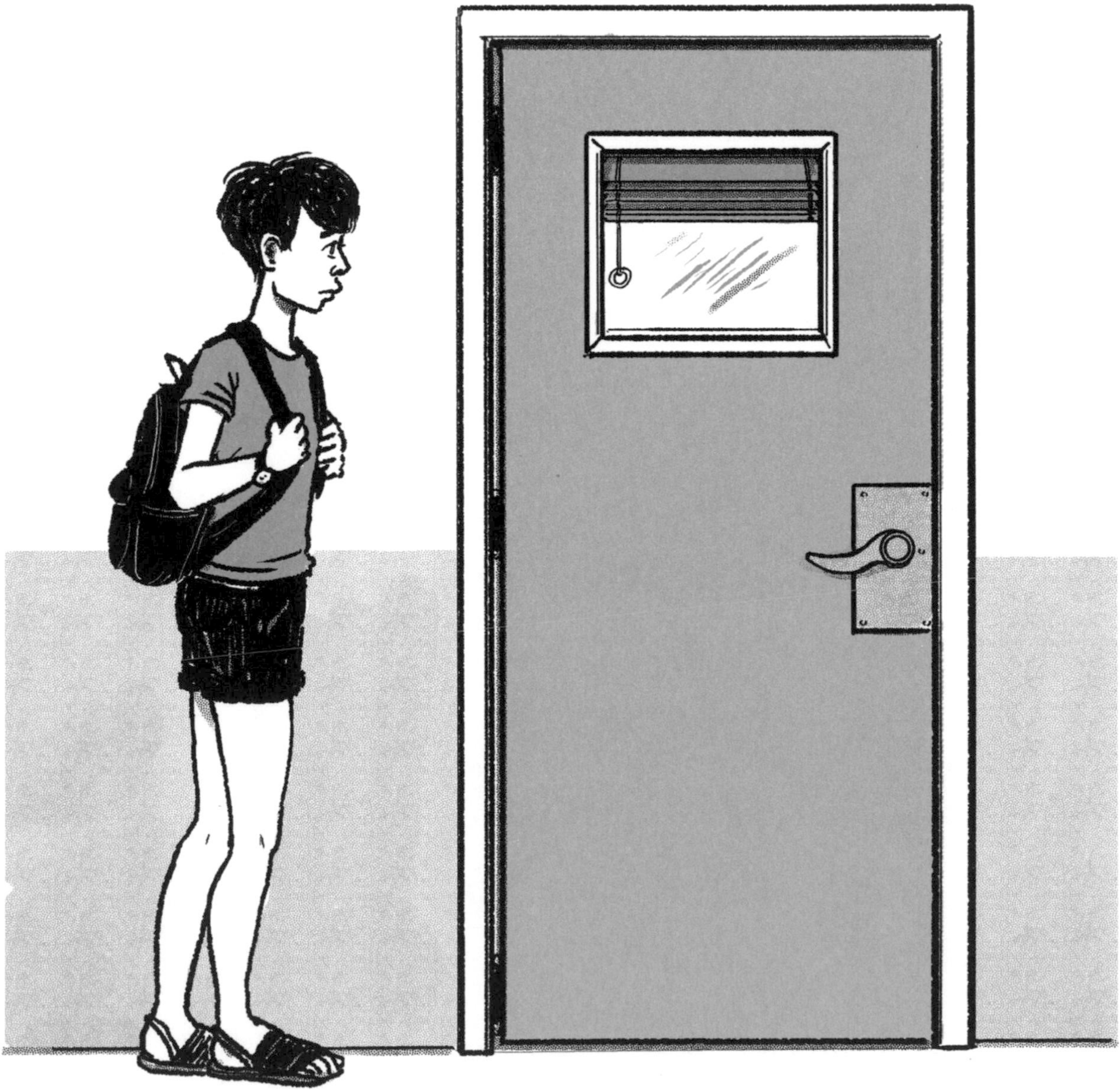

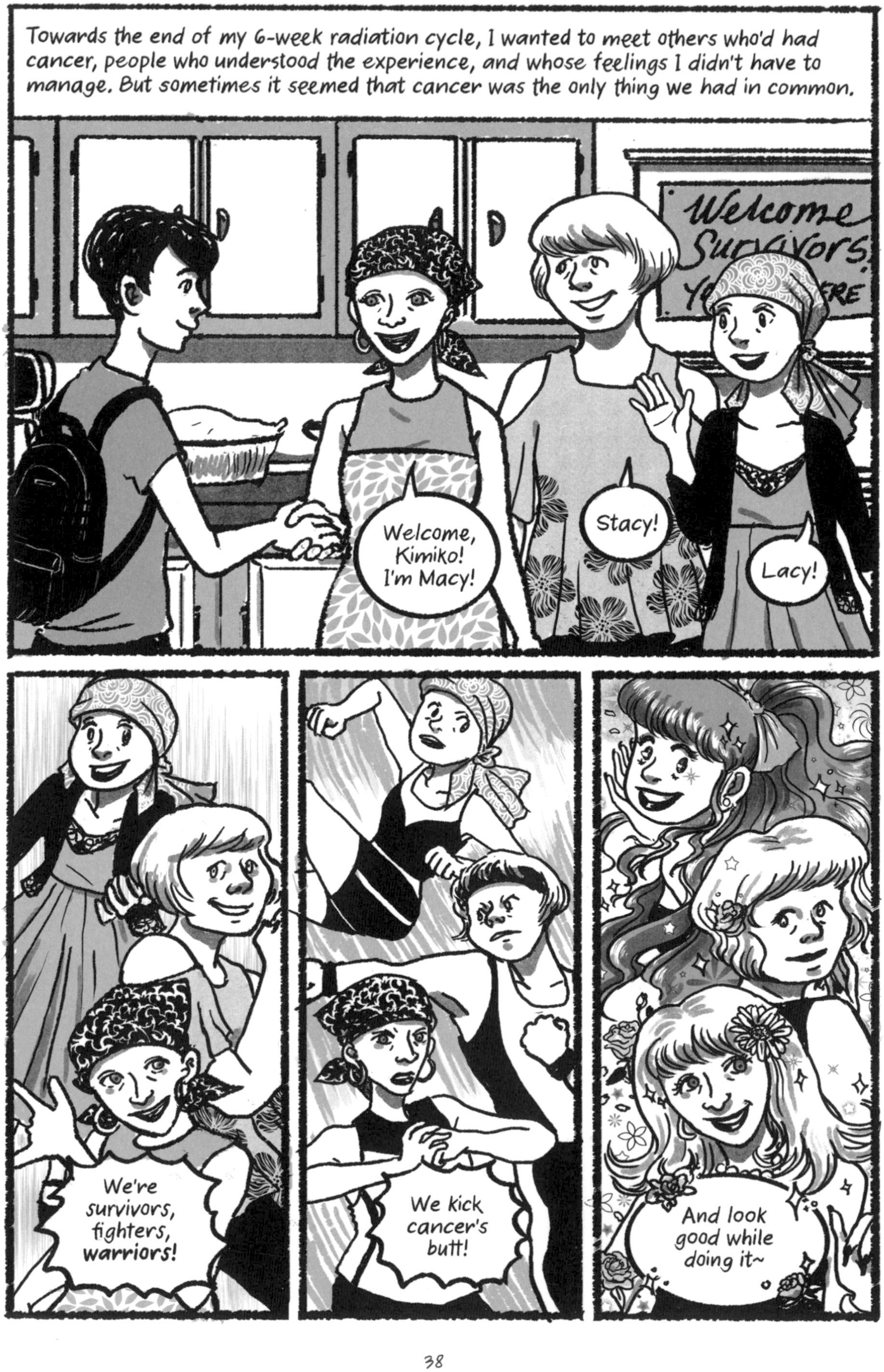
Towards the end of my 6-week radiation cycle, I wanted to meet others who'd had cancer, people who understood the experience, and whose feelings I didn't have to manage. But sometimes it seemed that cancer was the only thing we had in common.
Welcome Survivors
Welcome, Kimiko! I'm Macy!
Stacy!
Lacy!
We're survivors, fighters, **warriors!**
We kick cancer's butt!
And look good while doing it~

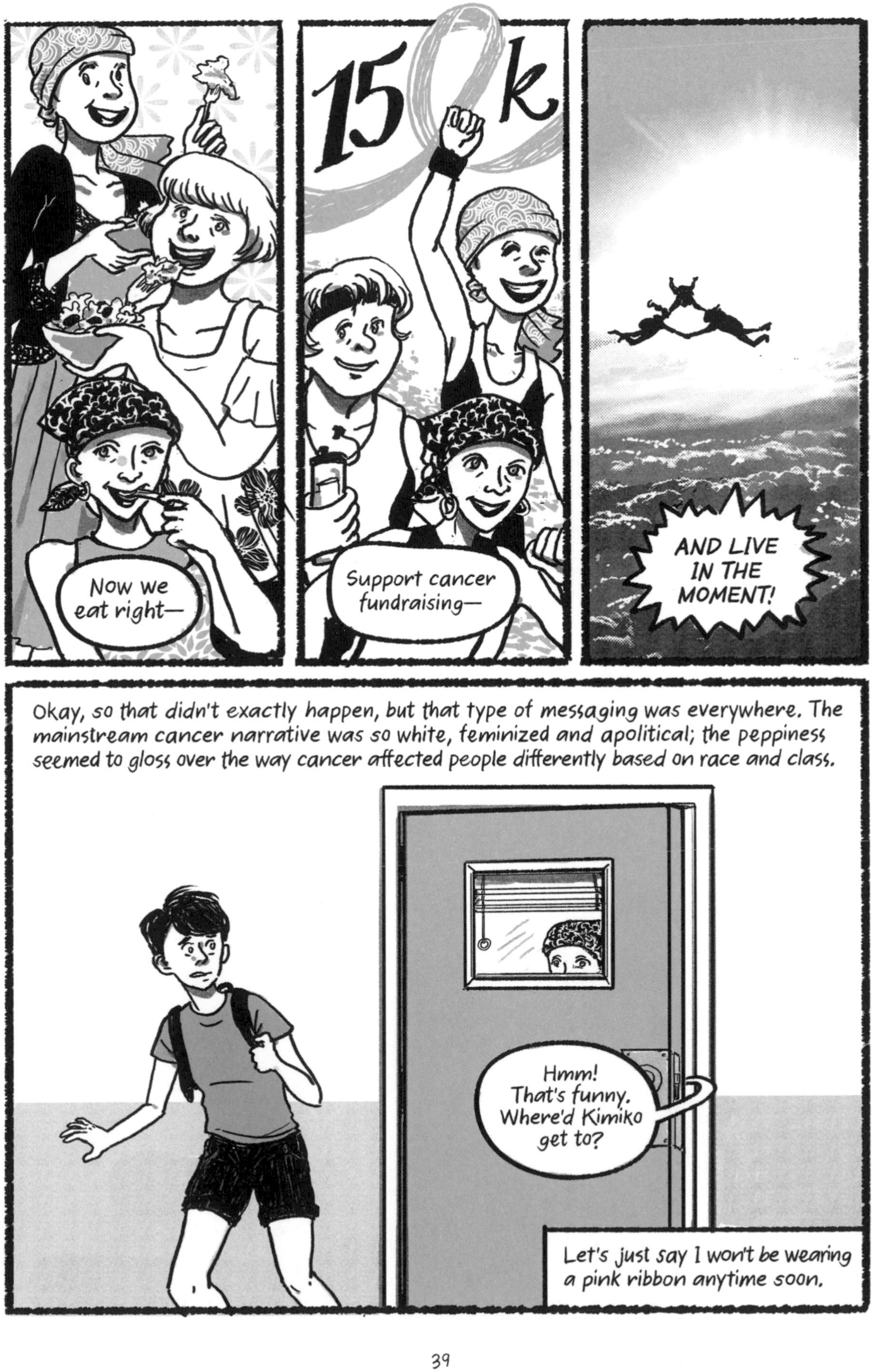
Now we eat right—
15 k
Support cancer fundraising—
AND LIVE IN THE MOMENT!
Okay, so that didn't exactly happen, but that type of messaging was everywhere. The mainstream cancer narrative was so white, feminized and apolitical; the peppiness seemed to gloss over the way cancer affected people differently based on race and class.
Hmm! That's funny. Where'd Kimiko get to?
Let's just say I won't be wearing a pink ribbon anytime soon.

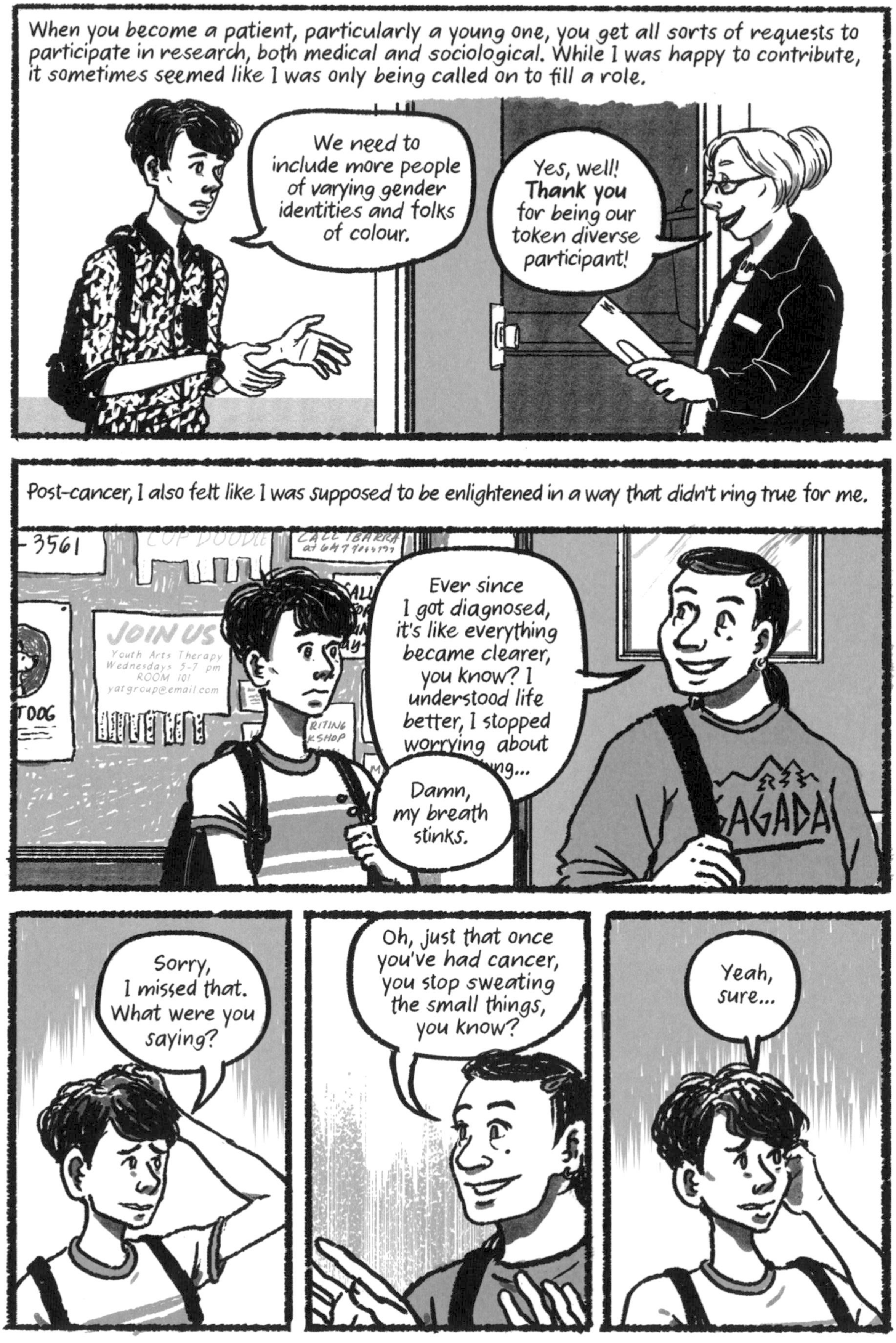
When you become a patient, particularly a young one, you get all sorts of requests to participate in research, both medical and sociological. While I was happy to contribute, it sometimes seemed like I was only being called on to fill a role.
We need to include more people of varying gender identities and folks of colour.
Yes, well! **Thank you** for being our token diverse participant!
Post-cancer, I also felt like I was supposed to be enlightened in a way that didn't ring true for me.
-3561
JOIN US
Youth Arts Therapy
Wednesdays 5-7 pm
ROOM 101
yatgroup@email.com
Ever since I got diagnosed, it's like everything became clearer, you know? I understood life better, I stopped worrying about
Damn, my breath stinks.
Sorry, I missed that. What were you saying?
Oh, just that once you've had cancer, you stop sweating the small things, you know?
Yeah, sure...

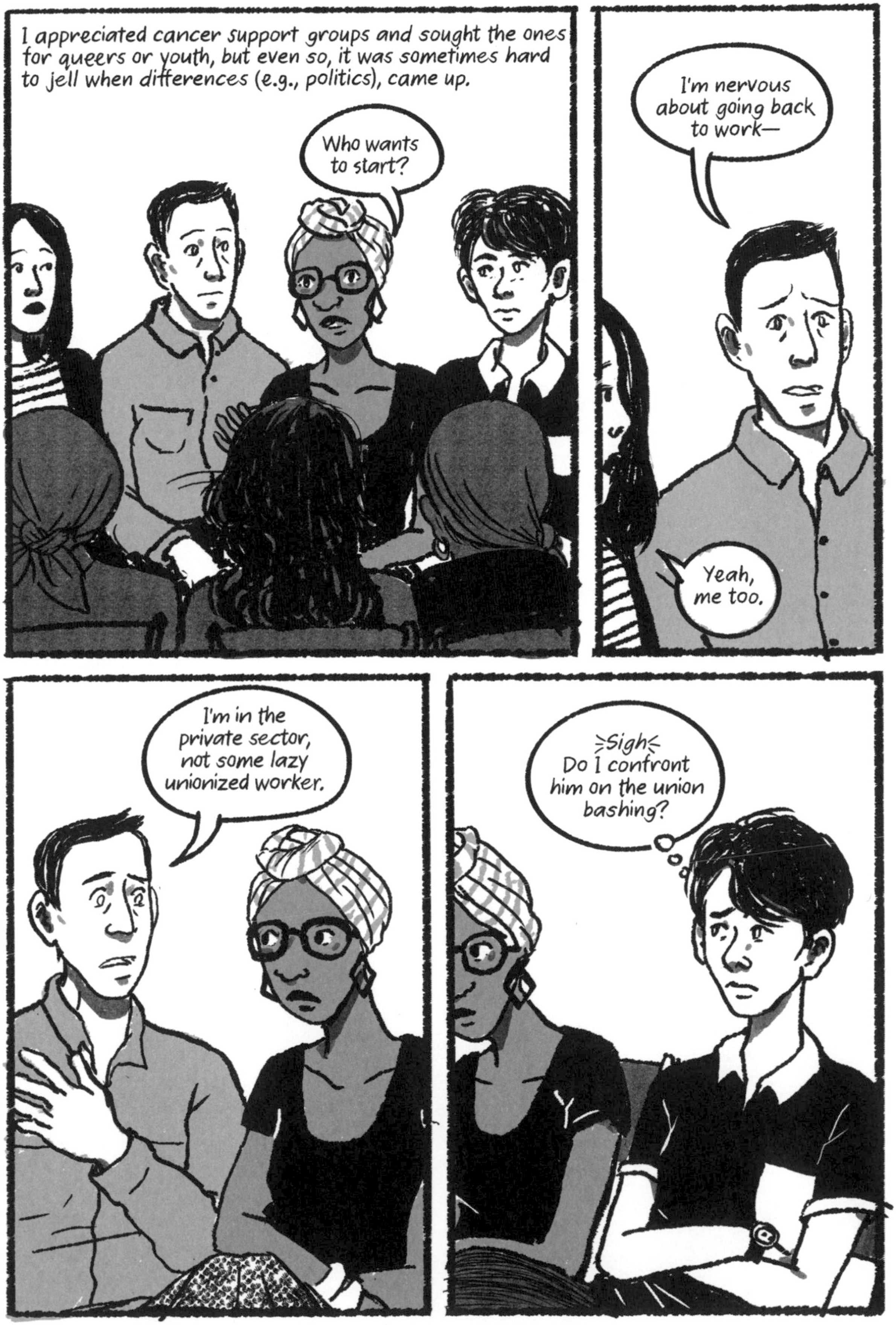
I appreciated cancer support groups and sought the ones for queers or youth, but even so, it was sometimes hard to jell when differences (e.g., politics), came up.
Who wants to start?
I'm nervous about going back to work—
Yeah, me too.
I'm in the private sector, not some lazy unionized worker.
Sigh
Do I confront him on the union bashing?

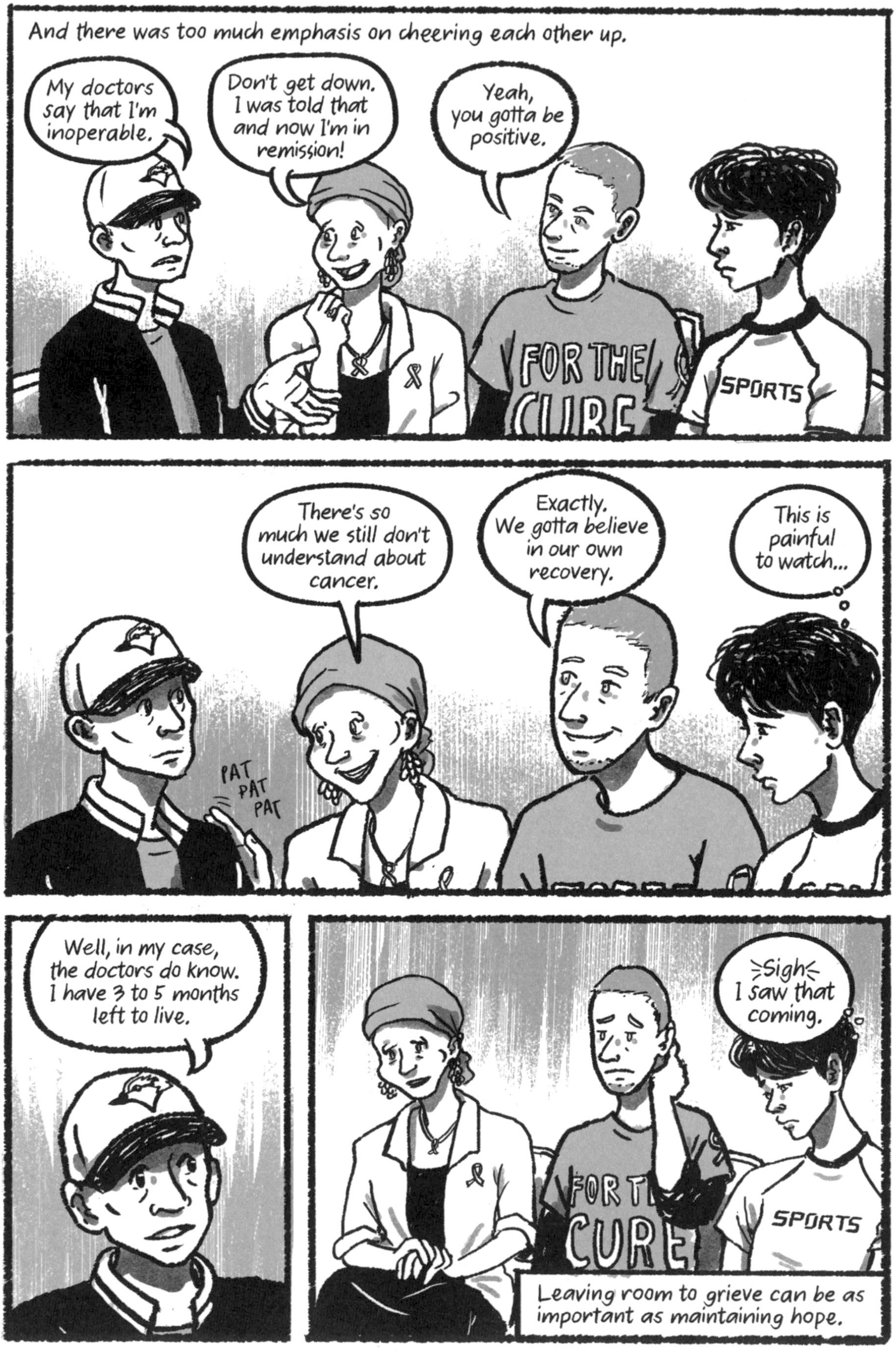
And there was too much emphasis on cheering each other up.
My doctors say that I'm inoperable.
Don't get down. I was told that and now I'm in remission!
Yeah, you gotta be positive.
FOR THE CURE
SPORTS
There's so much we still don't understand about cancer.
Exactly. We gotta believe in our own recovery.
This is painful to watch...
PAT PAT PAT
Well, in my case, the doctors do know. I have 3 to 5 months left to live.
Sigh I saw that coming.
FOR THE CURE
SPORTS
Leaving room to grieve can be as important as maintaining hope.

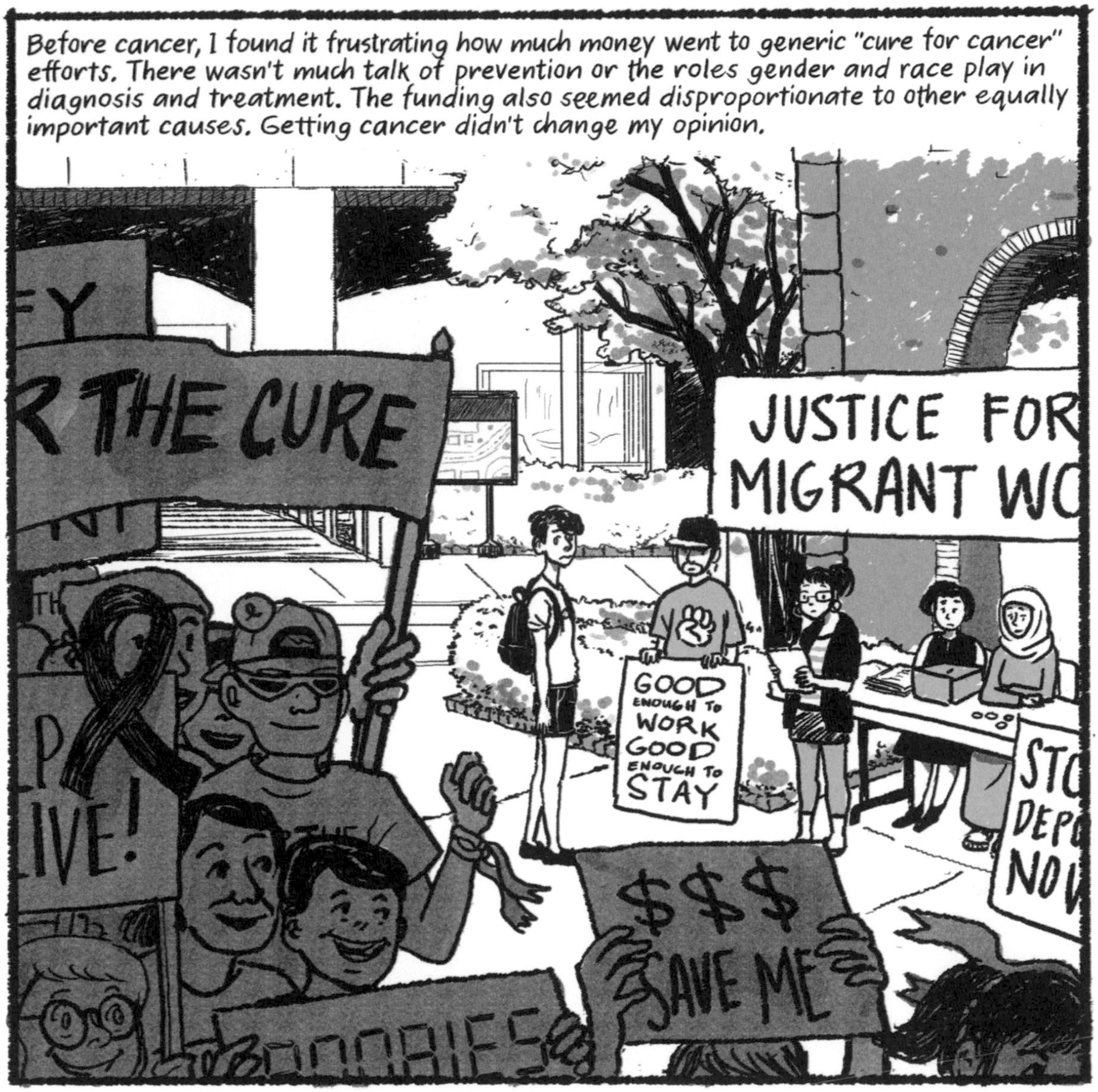
Before cancer, I found it frustrating how much money went to generic "cure for cancer" efforts. There wasn't much talk of prevention or the roles gender and race play in diagnosis and treatment. The funding also seemed disproportionate to other equally important causes. Getting cancer didn't change my opinion.
THE CURE
JUSTICE FOR
GOOD ENOUGH TO WORK GOOD ENOUGH TO STAY
$$$ SAVE ME

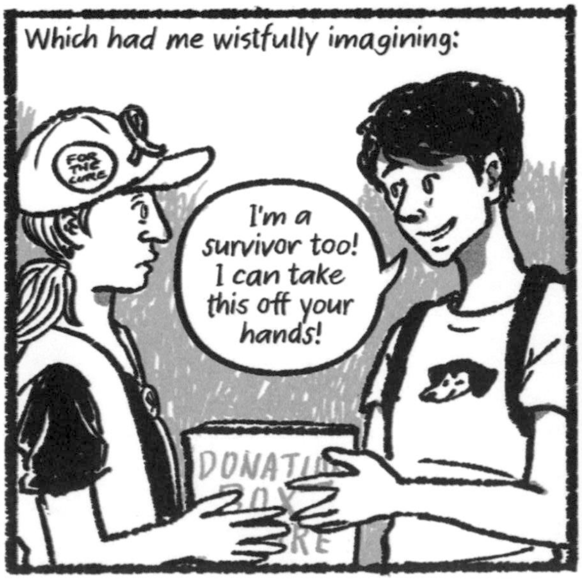
Which had me wistfully imagining:
FOR THE CURE
I'm a survivor too! I can take this off your hands!

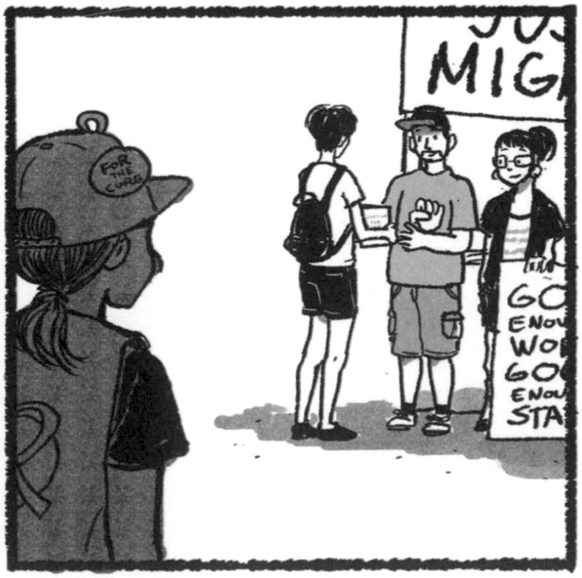
FOR THE CURE

But there were some perks to being in the cancer club.

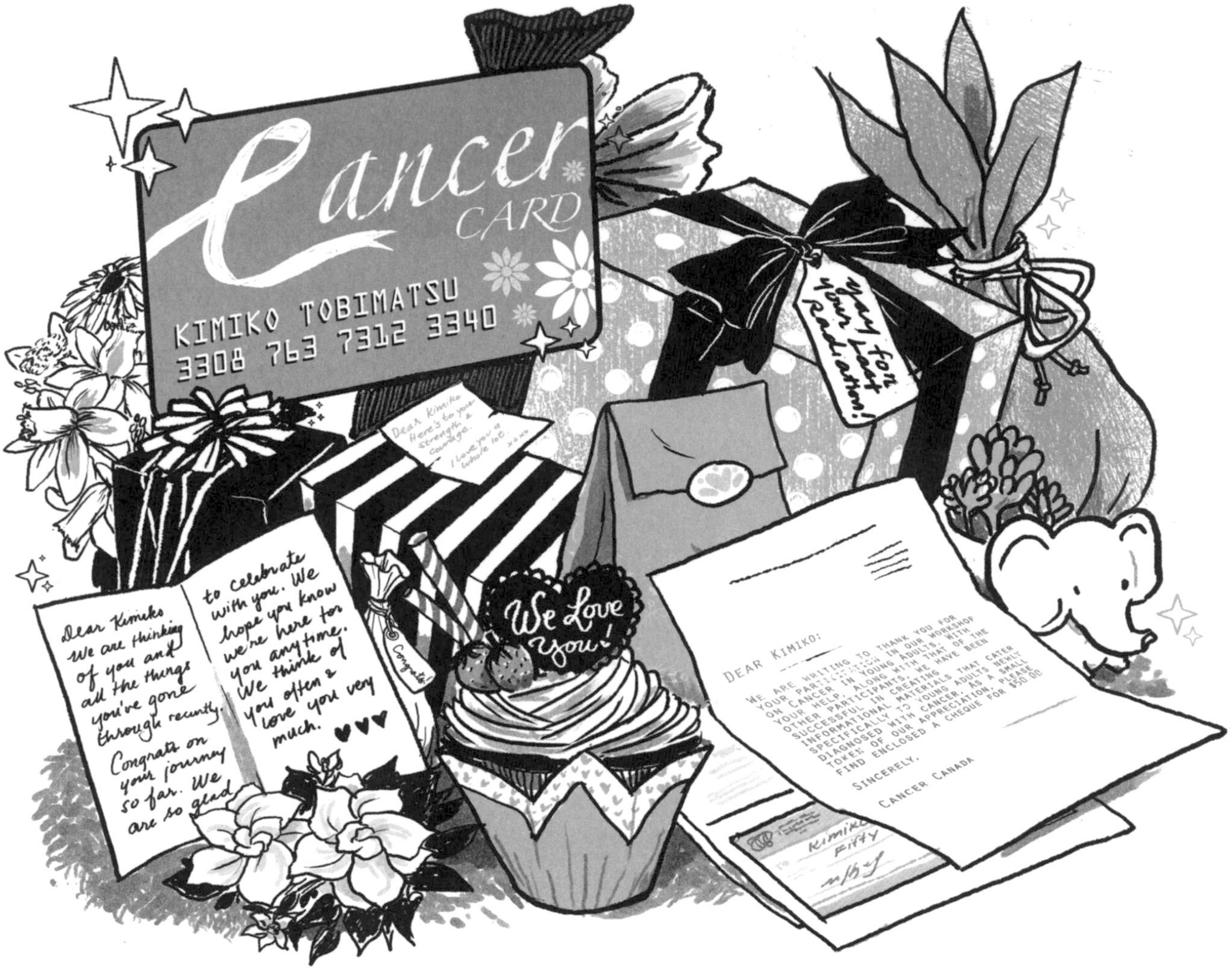
Cancer CARD
KIMIKO TOBIMATSU
3308 763 7312 3340
Yay for your last radiation!
Dear Kimiko Here's to your strength & courage. I love you a whole lot. xoxo
Dear Kimiko We are thinking of you and all the things you've gone through recently. Congrats on your journey so far. We are so glad
to celebrate with you. We hope you know we're here for you anytime. We think of you often & love you very much. ♥♥♥
Congrats
We Love You!
DEAR KIMIKO:
WE ARE WRITING TO THANK YOU FOR YOUR PARTICIPATION IN OUR WORKSHOP ON CANCER IN YOUNG ADULTS. WITH YOUR HELP, ALONG WITH THAT OF THE OTHER PARTICIPANTS, WE HAVE BEEN SUCCESSFUL IN CREATING INFORMATIONAL MATERIALS THAT CATER SPECIFICALLY TO YOUNG ADULTS NEWLY DIAGNOSED WITH CANCER. AS A SMALL TOKEN OF OUR APPRECIATION, PLEASE FIND ENCLOSED A CHEQUE FOR $50.00
SINCERELY,
CANCER CANADA
Kimiko
Fifty

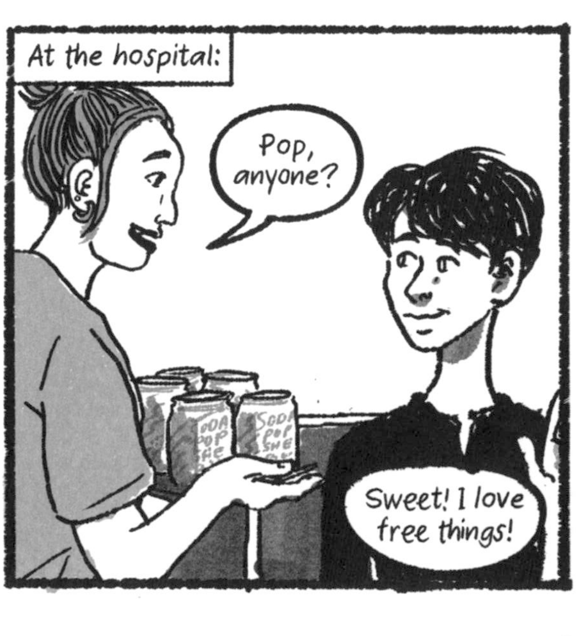
At the hospital:
Pop, anyone?
Sweet! I love free things!

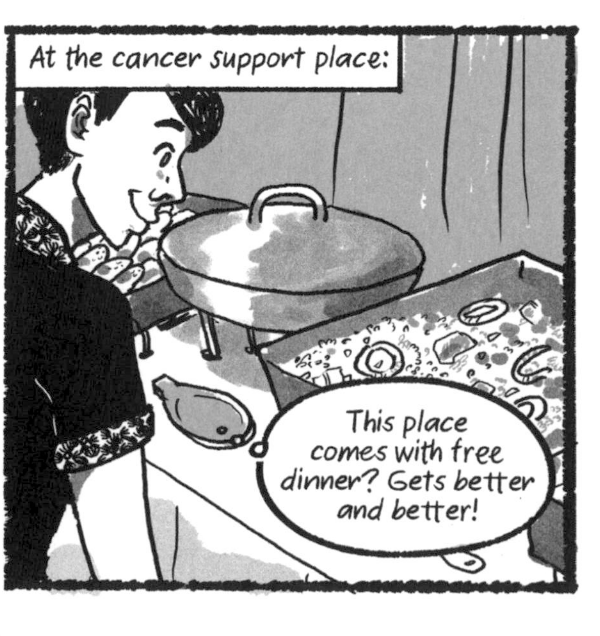
At the cancer support place:
This place comes with free dinner? Gets better and better!

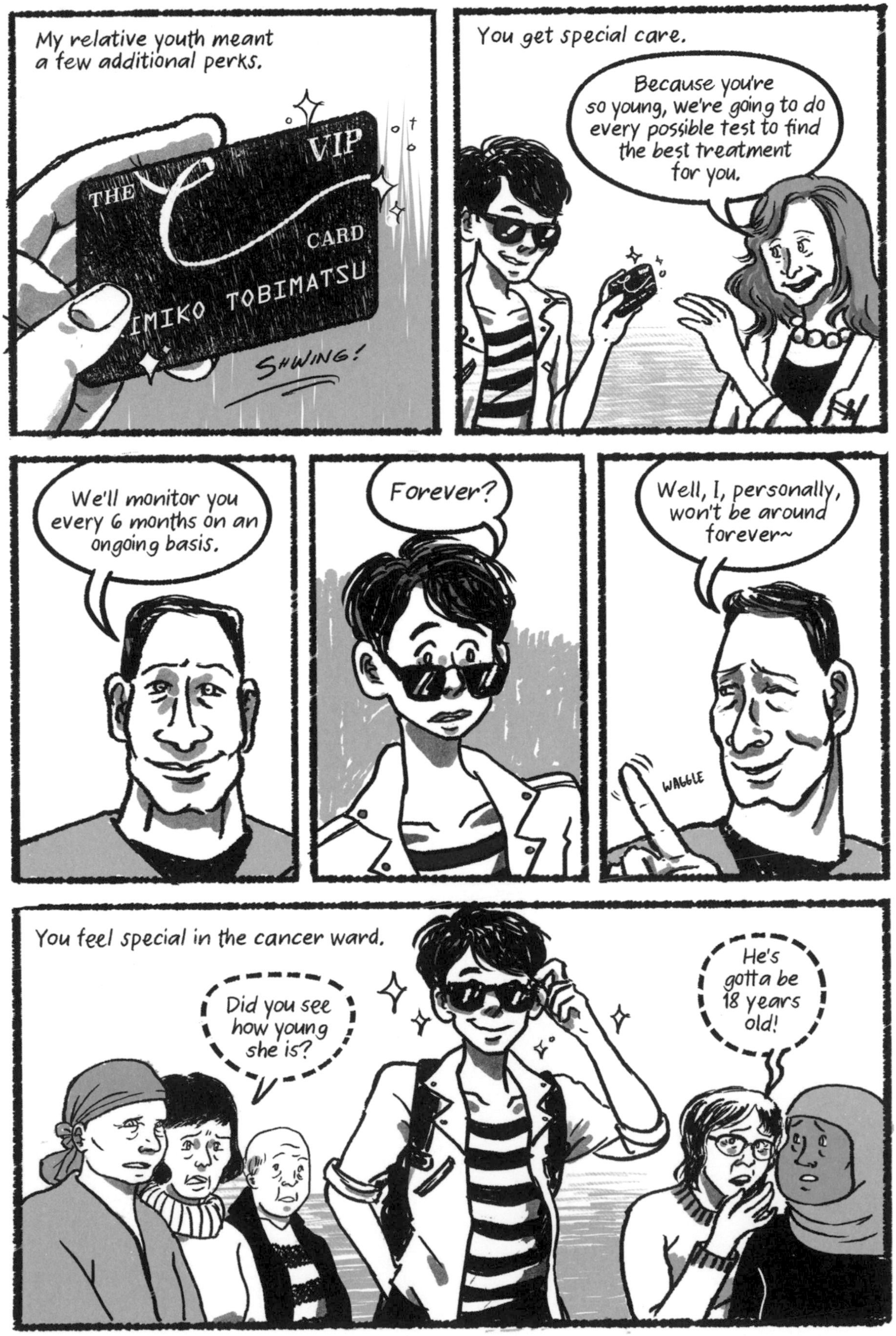
My relative youth meant a few additional perks.
THE VIP CARD
IMIKO TOBIMATSU
SHWING!
You get special care.
Because you're so young, we're going to do every possible test to find the best treatment for you.
We'll monitor you every 6 months on an ongoing basis.
Forever?
Well, I, personally, won't be around forever~
WAGGLE
You feel special in the cancer ward.
Did you see how young she is?
He's gotta be 18 years old!

THE IMPACT

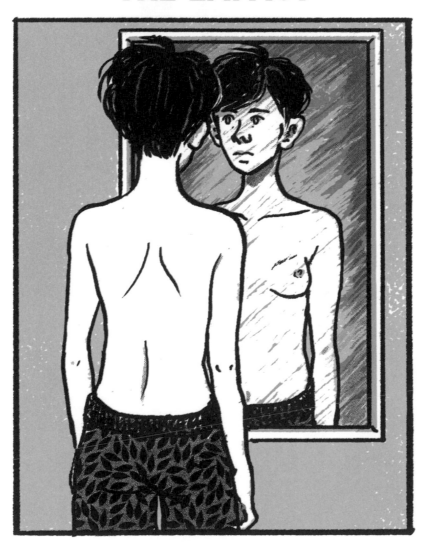

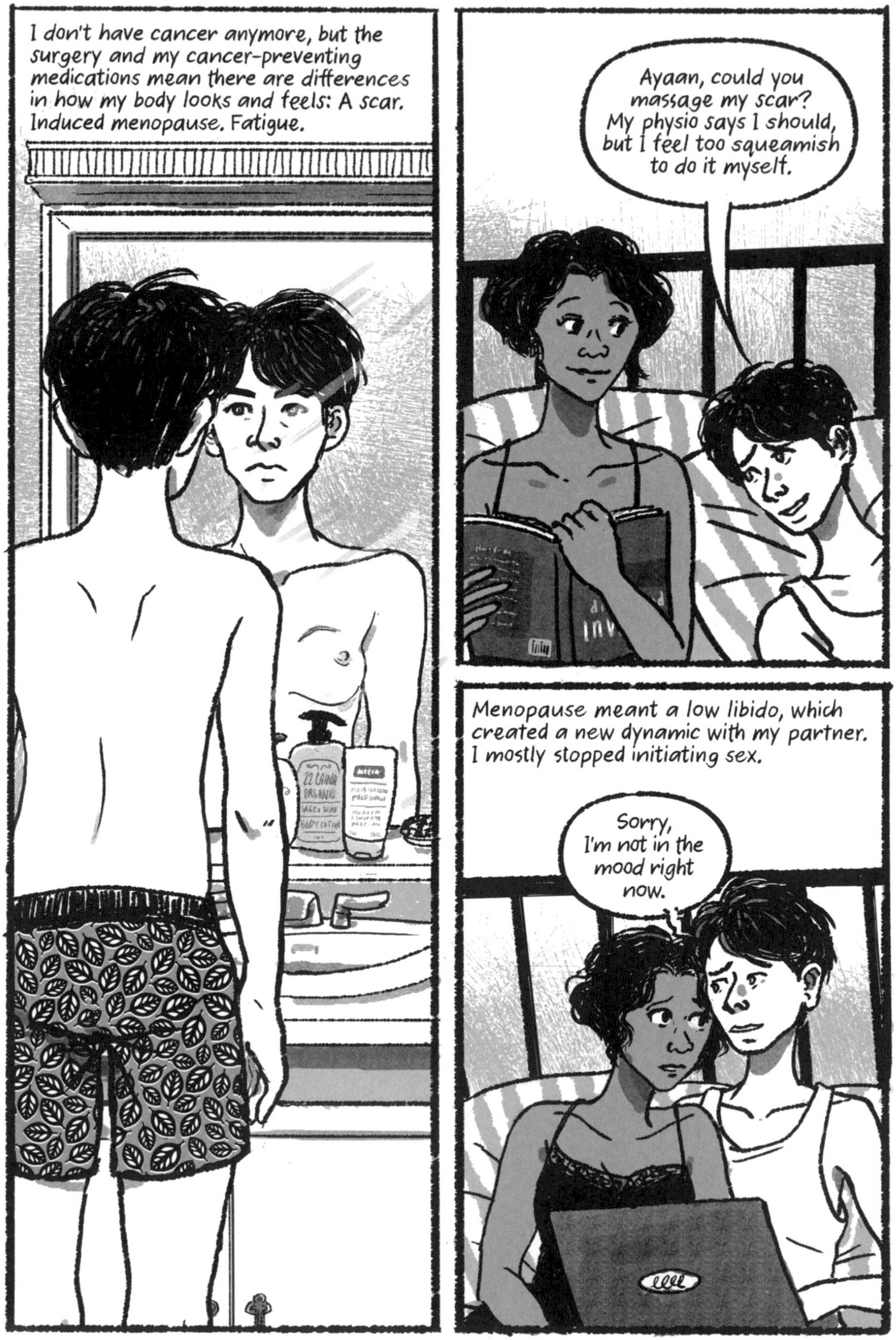
I don't have cancer anymore, but the surgery and my cancer-preventing medications mean there are differences in how my body looks and feels: A scar. Induced menopause. Fatigue.
Ayaan, could you massage my scar? My physio says I should, but I feel too squeamish to do it myself.
Menopause meant a low libido, which created a new dynamic with my partner. I mostly stopped initiating sex.
Sorry, I'm not in the mood right now.

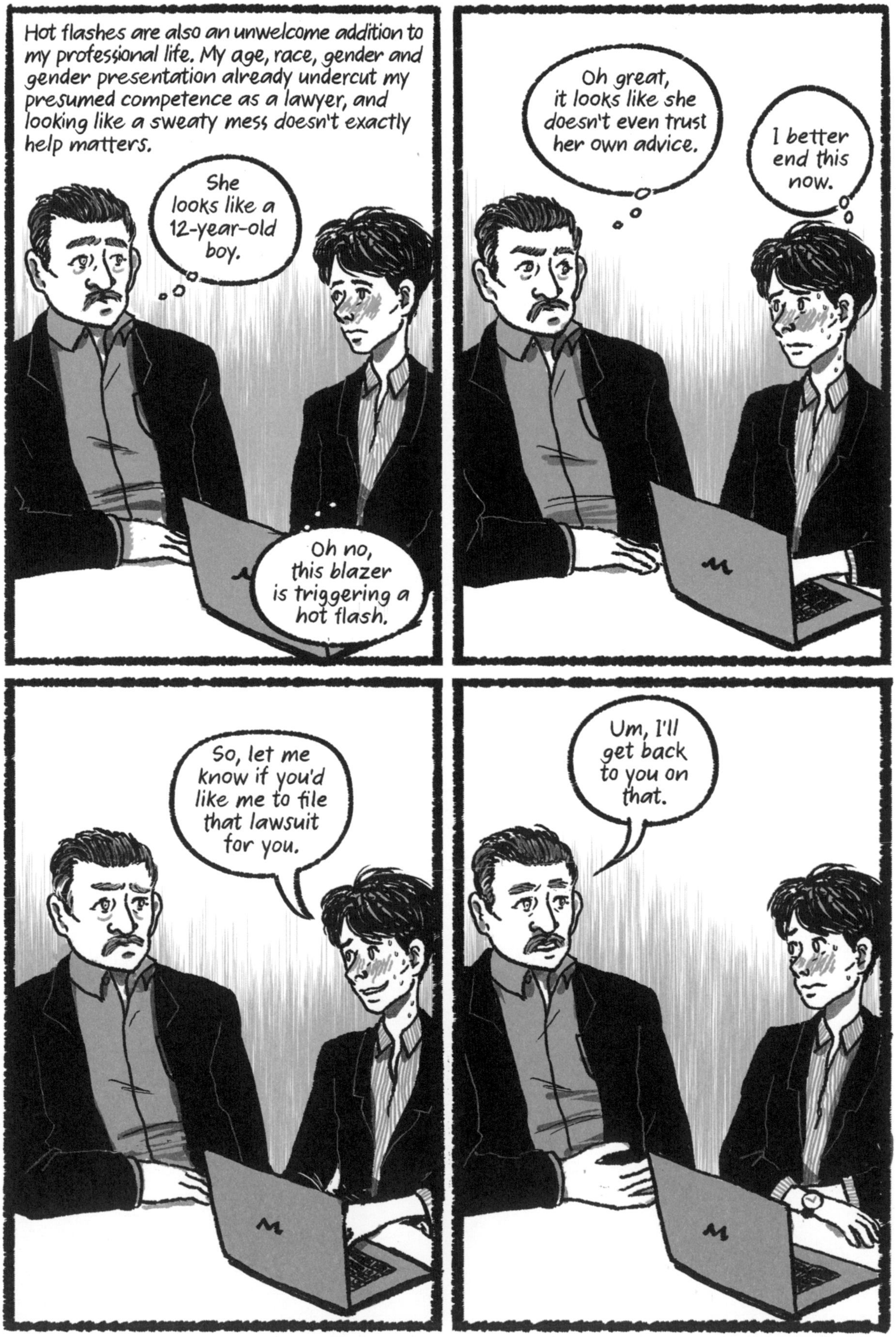
Hot flashes are also an unwelcome addition to my professional life. My age, race, gender and gender presentation already undercut my presumed competence as a lawyer, and looking like a sweaty mess doesn't exactly help matters.
She looks like a 12-year-old boy.
Oh no, this blazer is triggering a hot flash.
Oh great, it looks like she doesn't even trust her own advice.
I better end this now.
So, let me know if you'd like me to file that lawsuit for you.
Um, I'll get back to you on that.

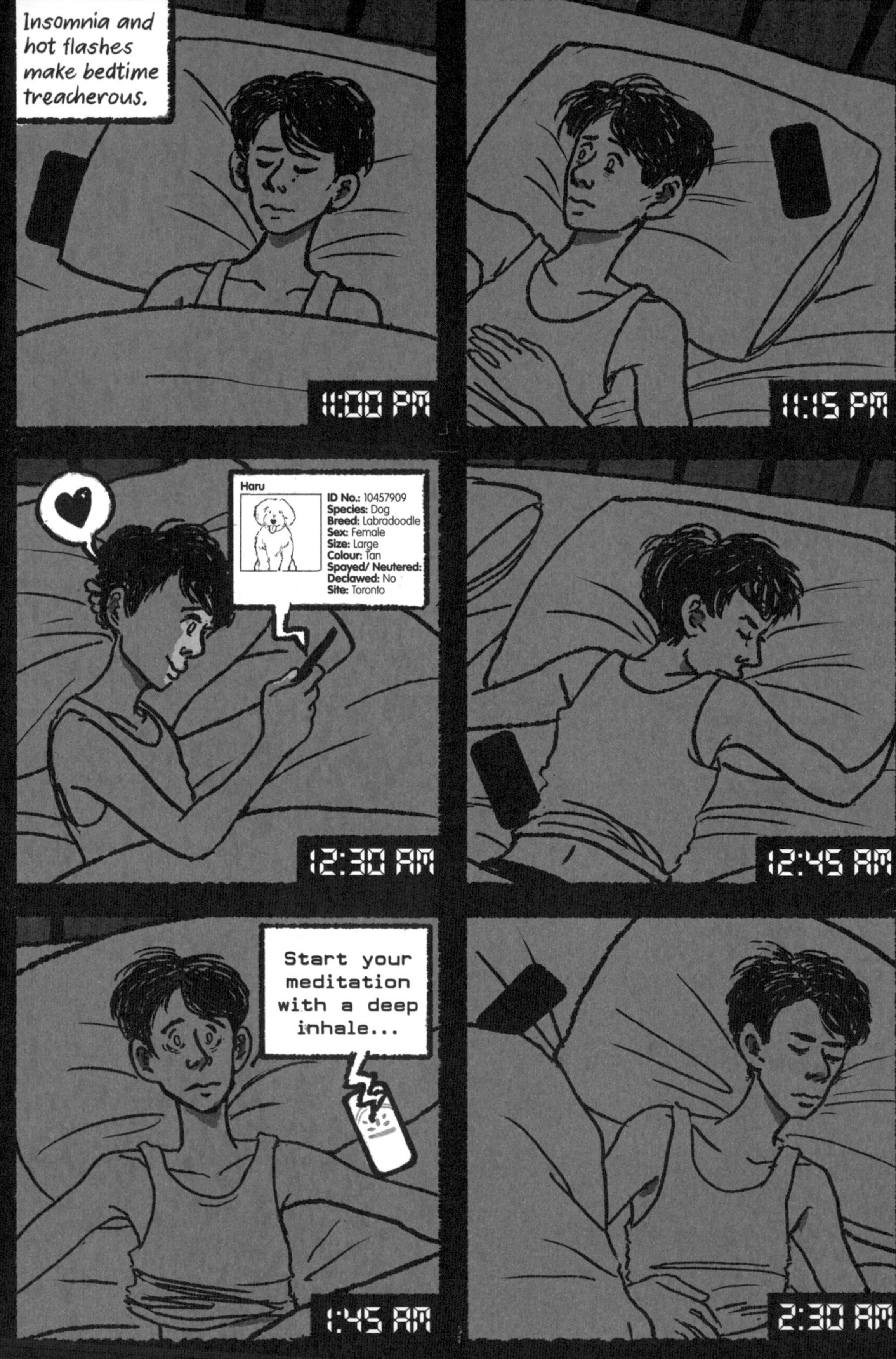

Insomnia and hot flashes make bedtime treacherous.
11:00 PM
11:15 PM
Haru
ID No.: 10457909
Species: Dog
Breed: Labradoodle
Sex: Female
Size: Large
Colour: Tan
Spayed/ Neutered:
Declawed: No
Site: Toronto
12:30 AM
12:45 AM
Start your meditation with a deep inhale...
1:45 AM
2:30 AM

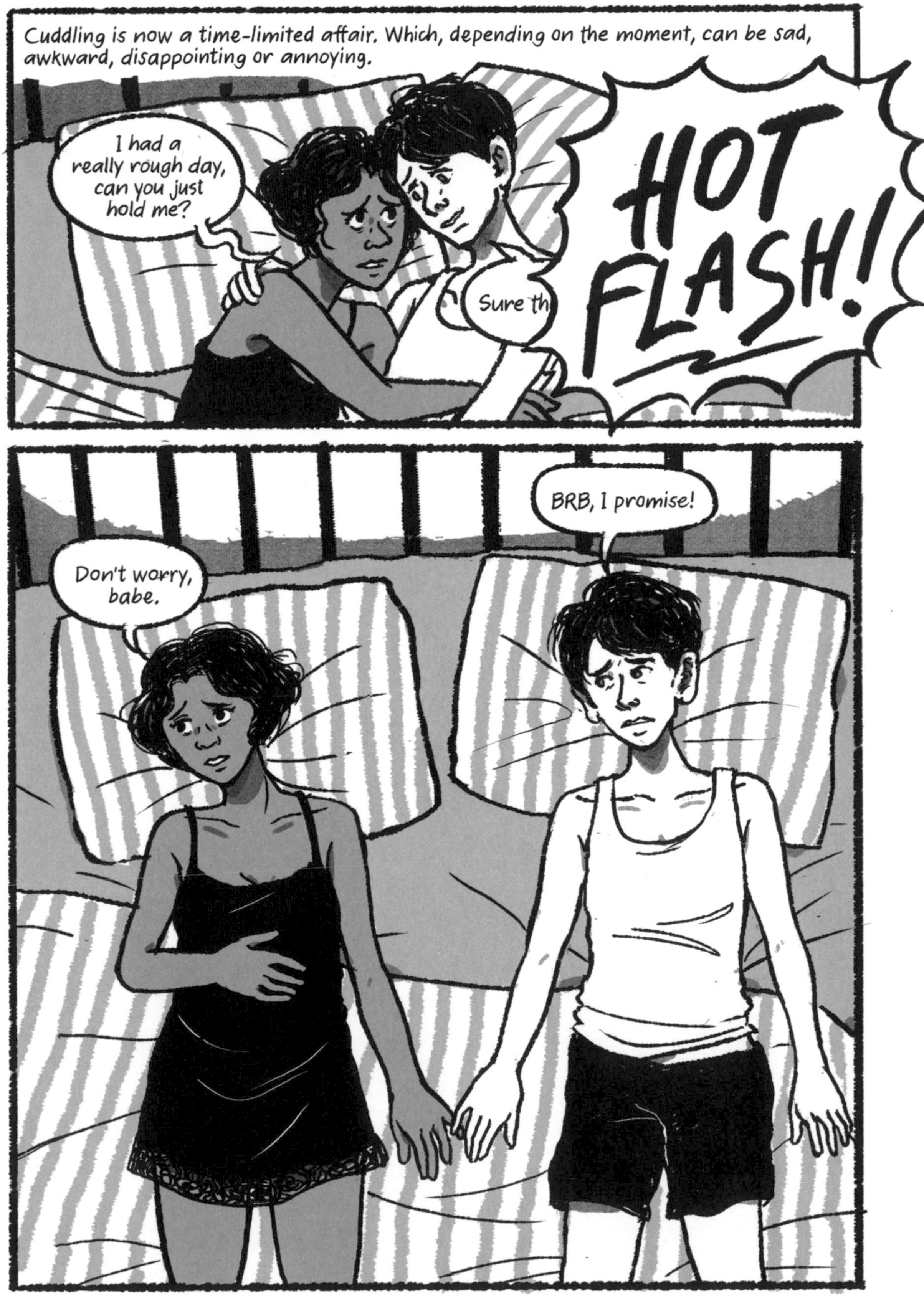
Cuddling is now a time-limited affair. Which, depending on the moment, can be sad, awkward, disappointing or annoying.
I had a really rough day, can you just hold me?
Sure th
HOT FLASH!!
Don't worry, babe.
BRB, I promise!

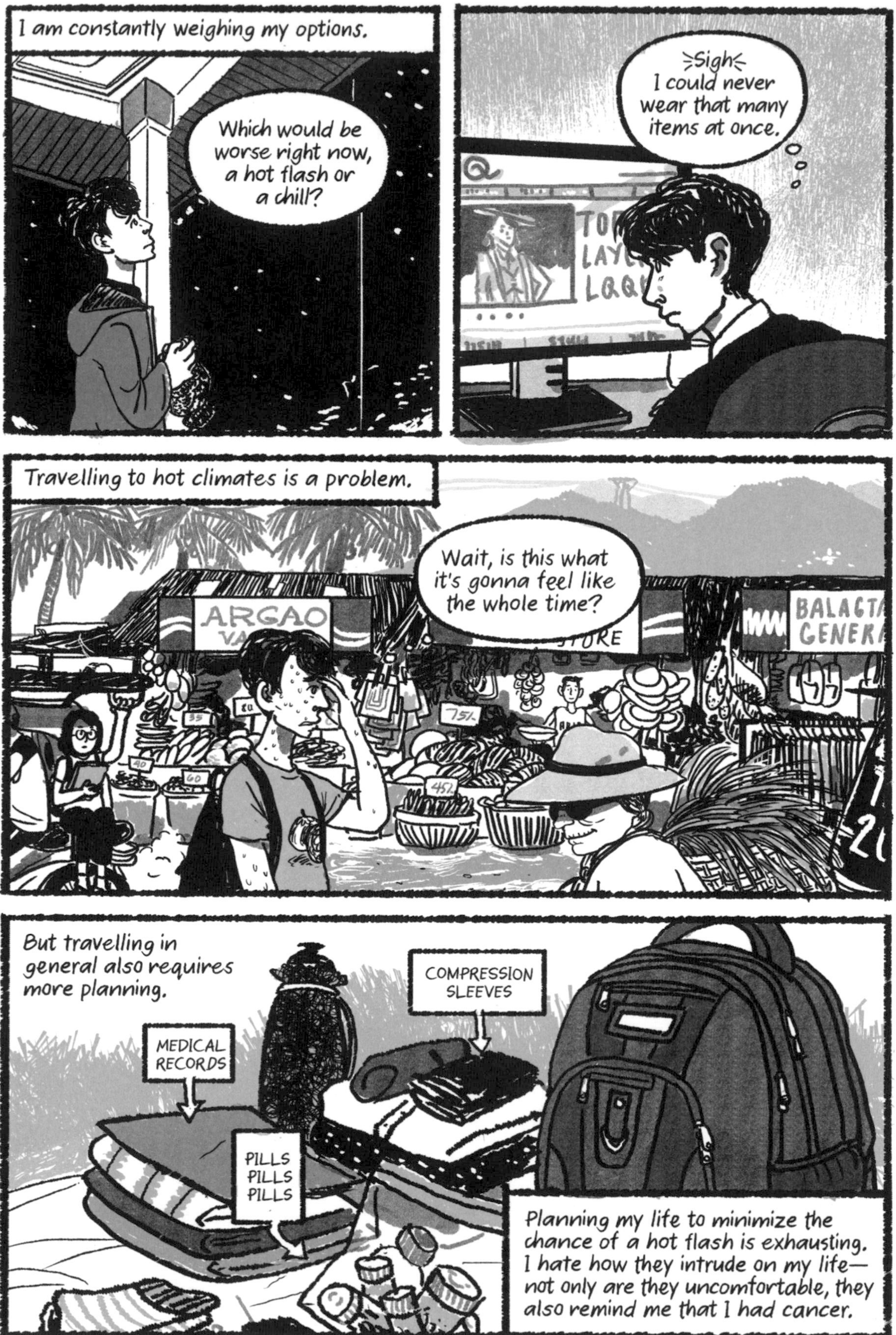
I am constantly weighing my options.
Which would be worse right now, a hot flash or a chill?
≥Sigh≤ I could never wear that many items at once.
Travelling to hot climates is a problem.
Wait, is this what it's gonna feel like the whole time?
ARGAO
But travelling in general also requires more planning.
COMPRESSION SLEEVES
MEDICAL RECORDS
PILLS PILLS PILLS
Planning my life to minimize the chance of a hot flash is exhausting. I hate how they intrude on my life—not only are they uncomfortable, they also remind me that I had cancer.

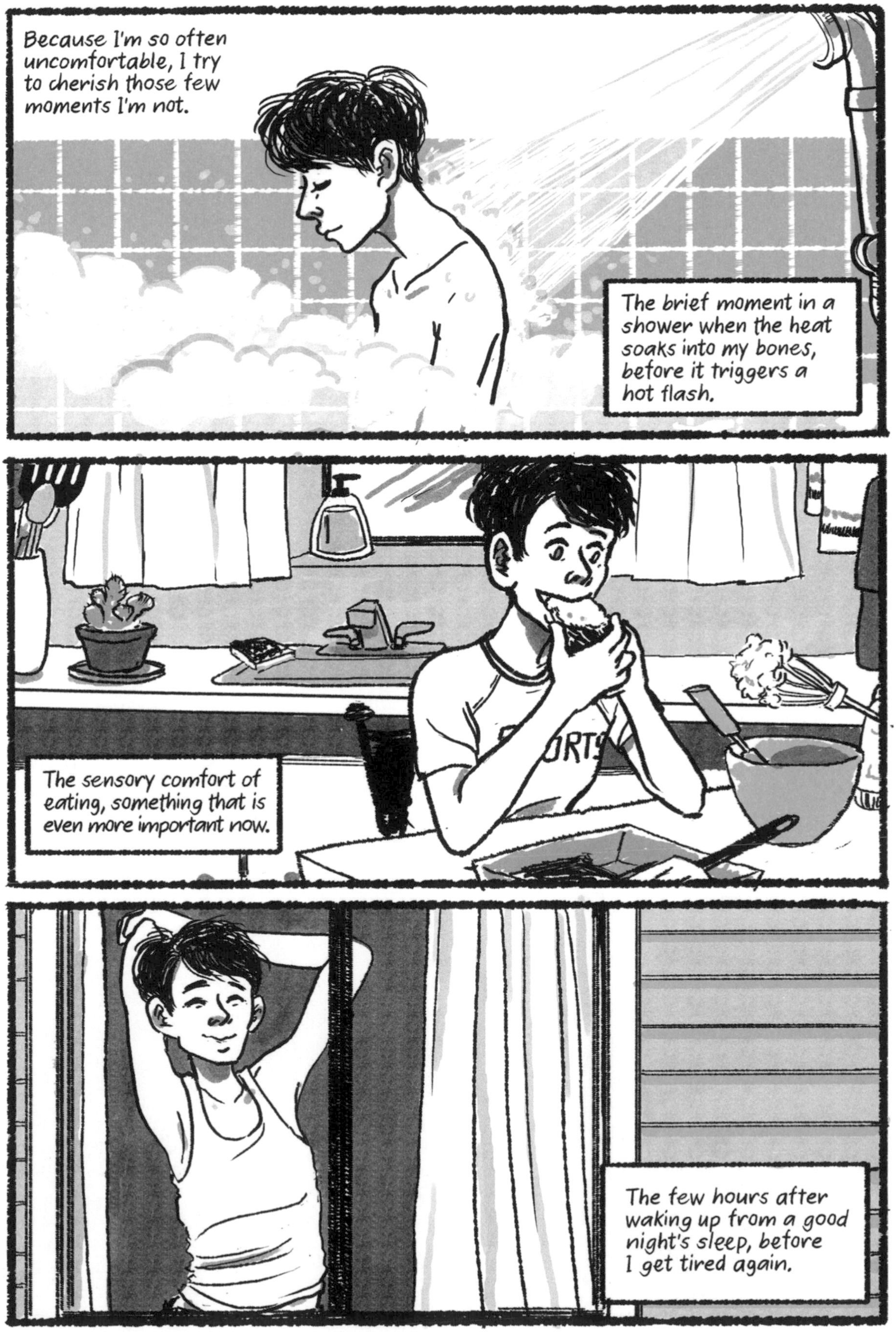
Because I'm so often uncomfortable, I try to cherish those few moments I'm not.
The brief moment in a shower when the heat soaks into my bones, before it triggers a hot flash.
The sensory comfort of eating, something that is even more important now.
The few hours after waking up from a good night's sleep, before I get tired again.

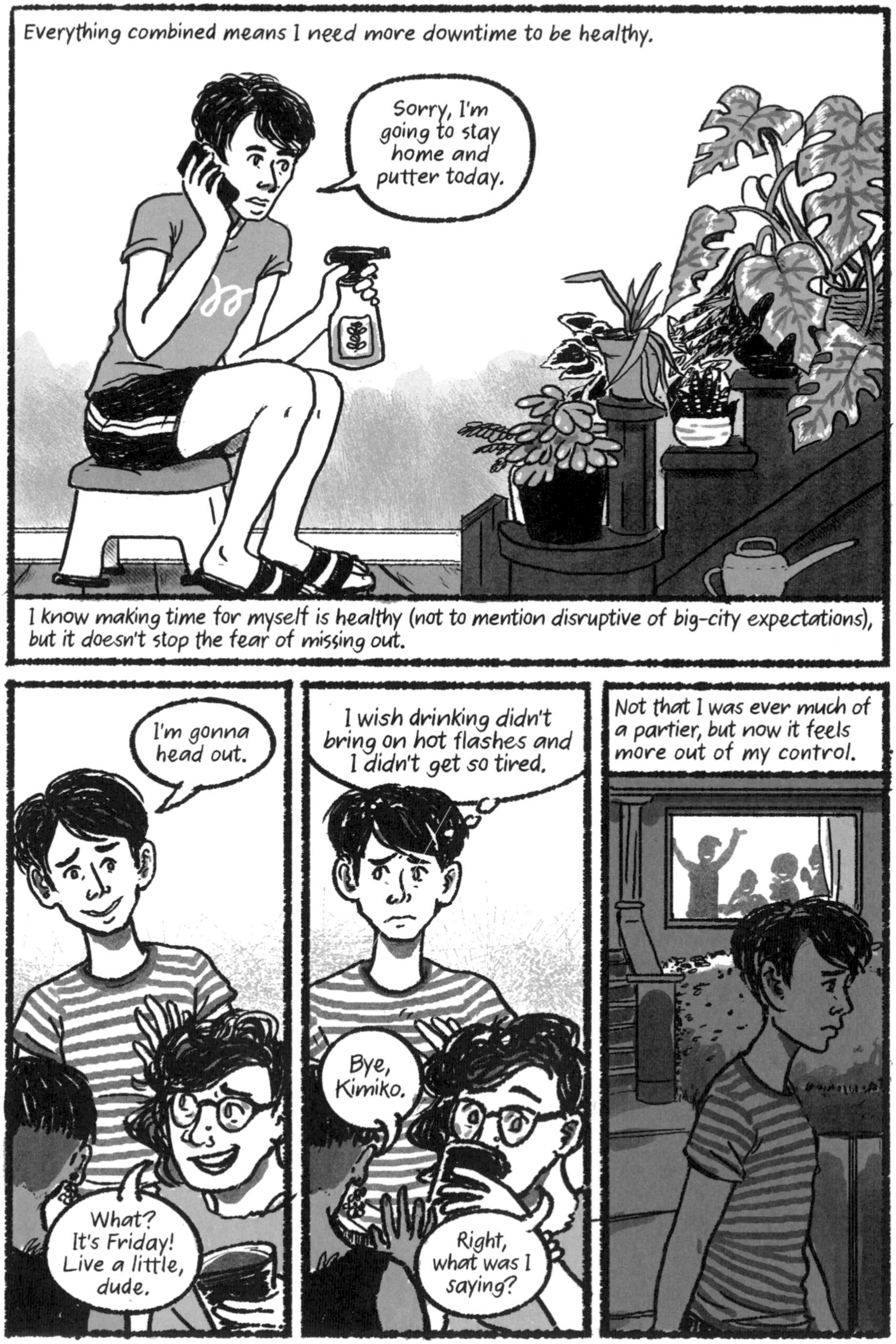
Everything combined means I need more downtime to be healthy.
Sorry, I'm going to stay home and putter today.
I know making time for myself is healthy (not to mention disruptive of big-city expectations), but it doesn't stop the fear of missing out.
I'm gonna head out.
What? It's Friday! Live a little, dude.
I wish drinking didn't bring on hot flashes and I didn't get so tired.
Bye, Kimiko.
Right, what was I saying?
Not that I was ever much of a partier, but now it feels more out of my control.

Searching for the perfect drugs to minimize symptoms is a constant struggle.

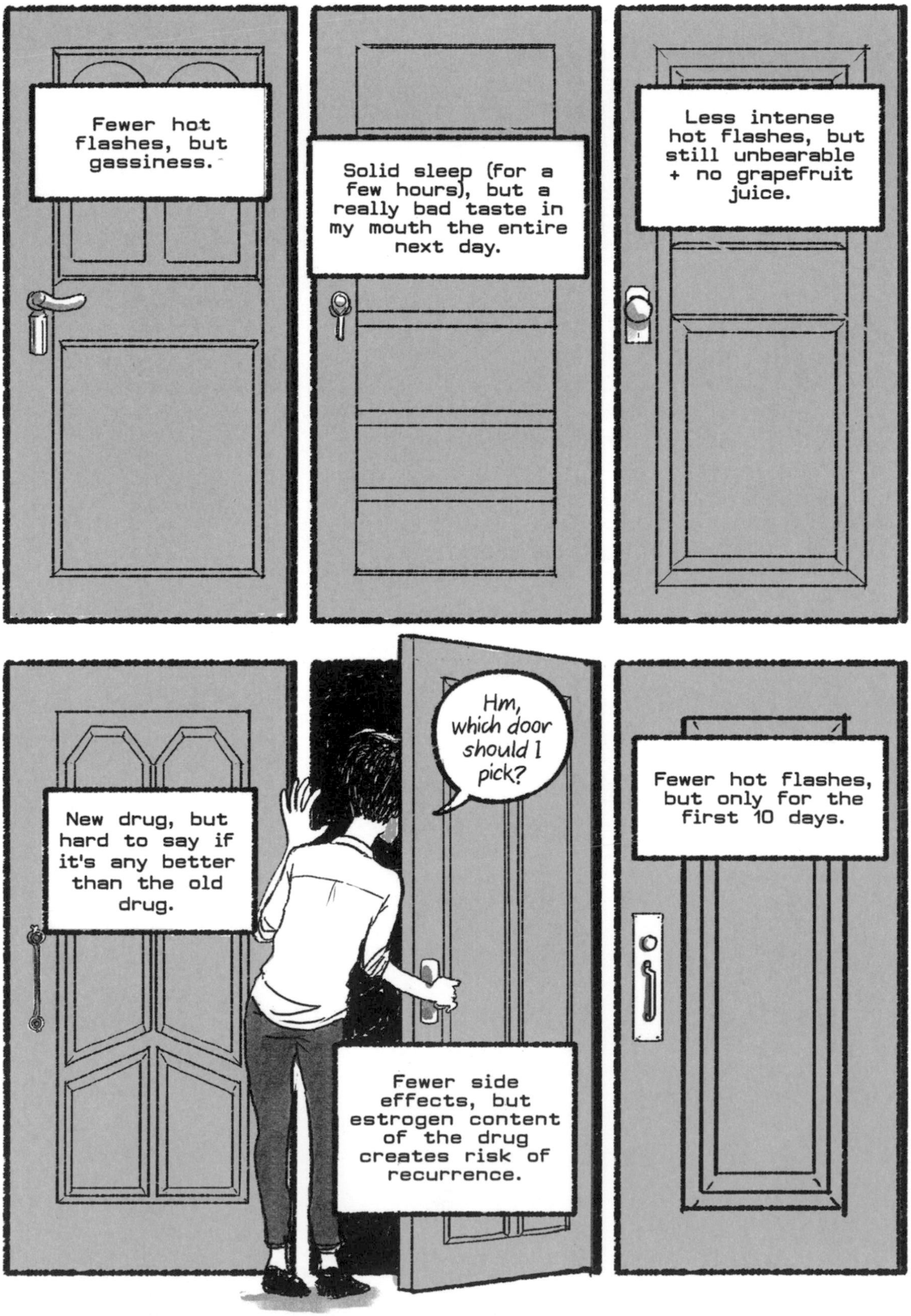

Fewer hot flashes, but gassiness.
Solid sleep (for a few hours), but a really bad taste in my mouth the entire next day.
Less intense hot flashes, but still unbearable + no grapefruit juice.
New drug, but hard to say if it's any better than the old drug.
Hm, which door should I pick?
Fewer side effects, but estrogen content of the drug creates risk of recurrence.
Fewer hot flashes, but only for the first 10 days.

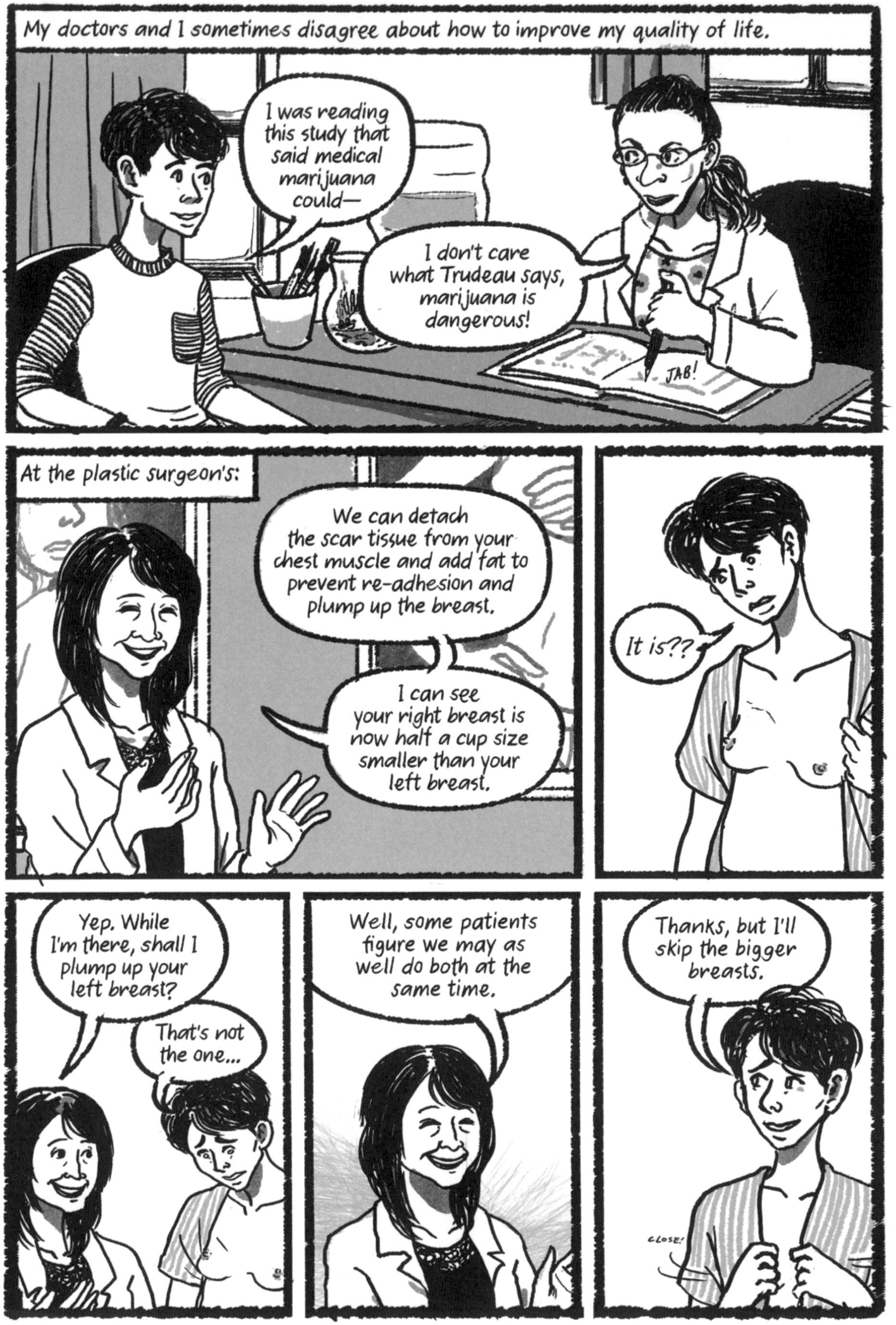
My doctors and I sometimes disagree about how to improve my quality of life.
I was reading this study that said medical marijuana could—
I don't care what Trudeau says, marijuana is dangerous!
JAB!
At the plastic surgeon's:
We can detach the scar tissue from your chest muscle and add fat to prevent re-adhesion and plump up the breast.
I can see your right breast is now half a cup size smaller than your left breast.
It is??
Yep. While I'm there, shall I plump up your left breast?
That's not the one...
Well, some patients figure we may as well do both at the same time.
Thanks, but I'll skip the bigger breasts.
CLOSE!

Even before cancer, mystery ailments could make my mind wander to worst-case scenarios. The difference now is that they don't seem so improbable.

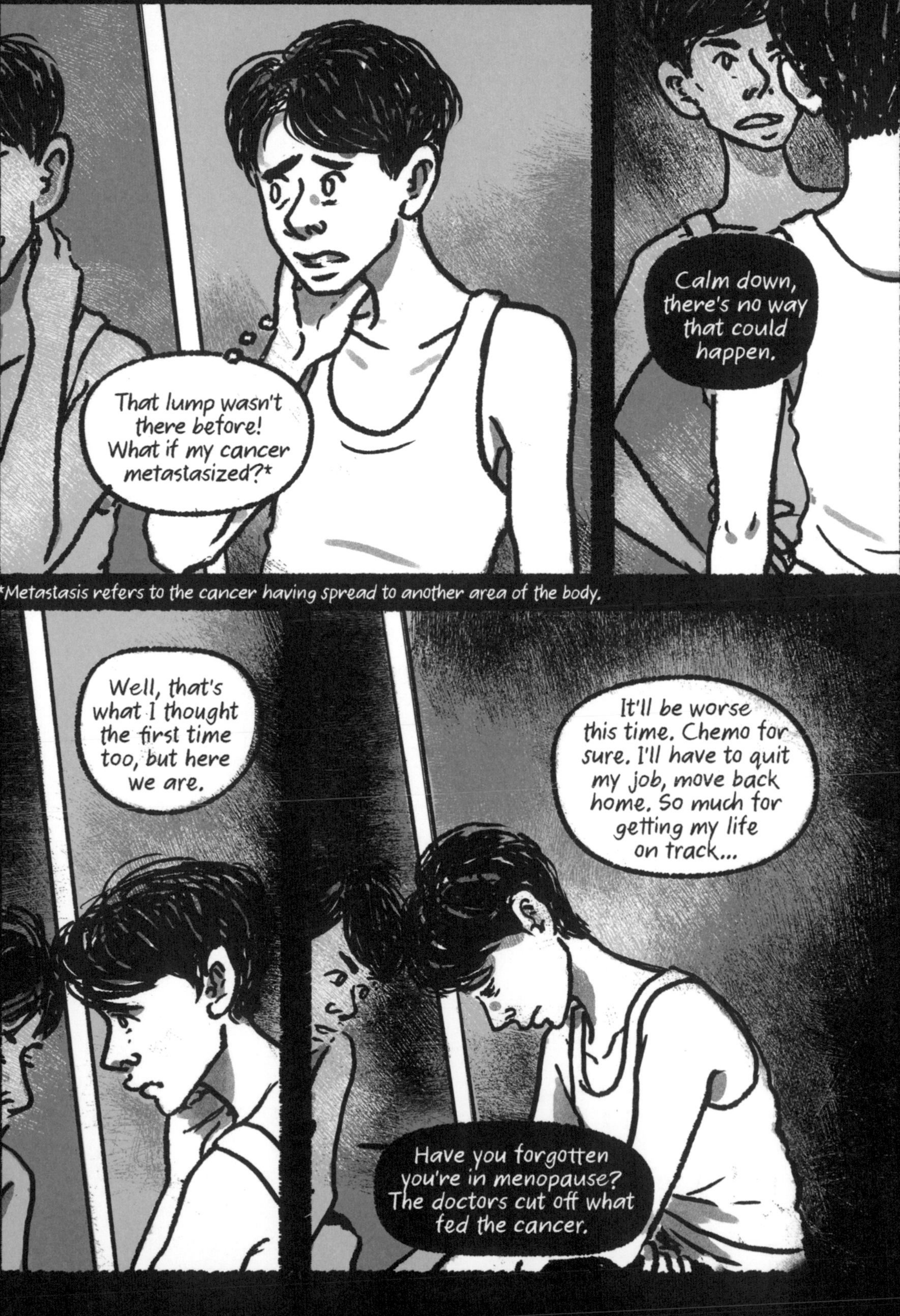

That lump wasn't there before! What if my cancer metastasized?*
Calm down, there's no way that could happen.
Well, that's what I thought the first time too, but here we are.
It'll be worse this time. Chemo for sure. I'll have to quit my job, move back home. So much for getting my life on track...
Have you forgotten you're in menopause? The doctors cut off what fed the cancer.

*Metastasis refers to the cancer having spread to another area of the body.

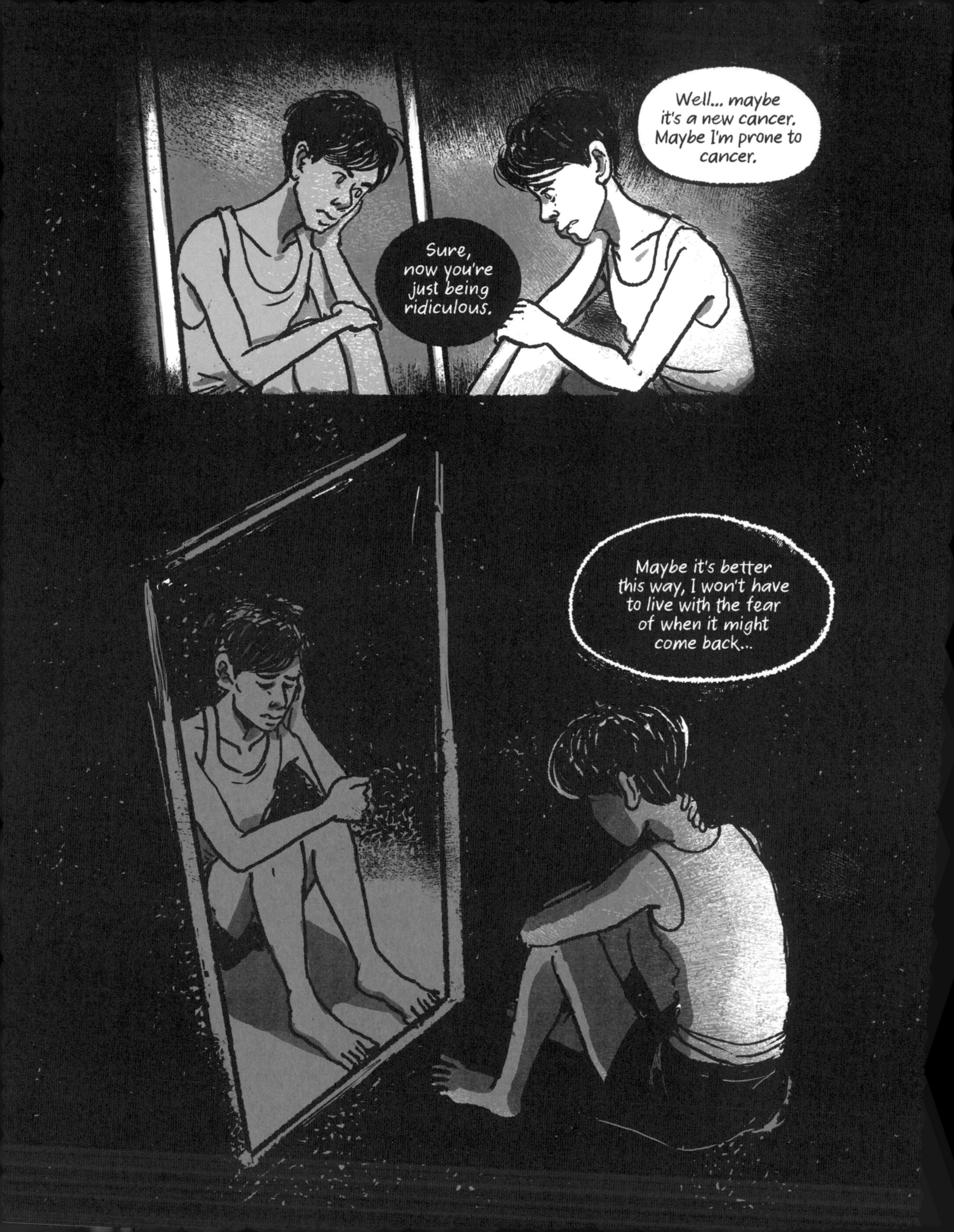
Well... maybe it's a new cancer. Maybe I'm prone to cancer.
Sure, now you're just being ridiculous.
Maybe it's better this way, I won't have to live with the fear of when it might come back...

THE NEW NORMAL

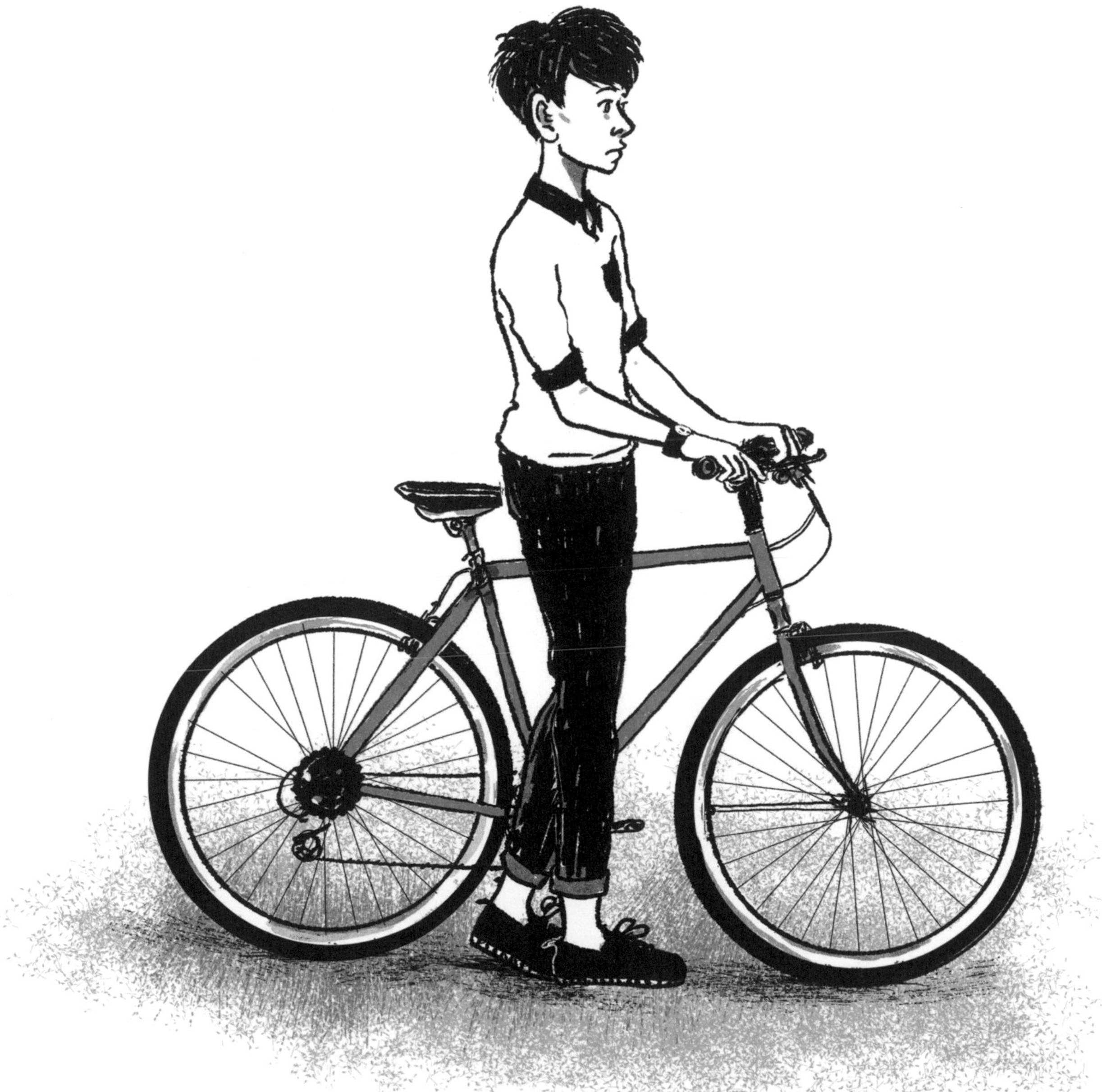

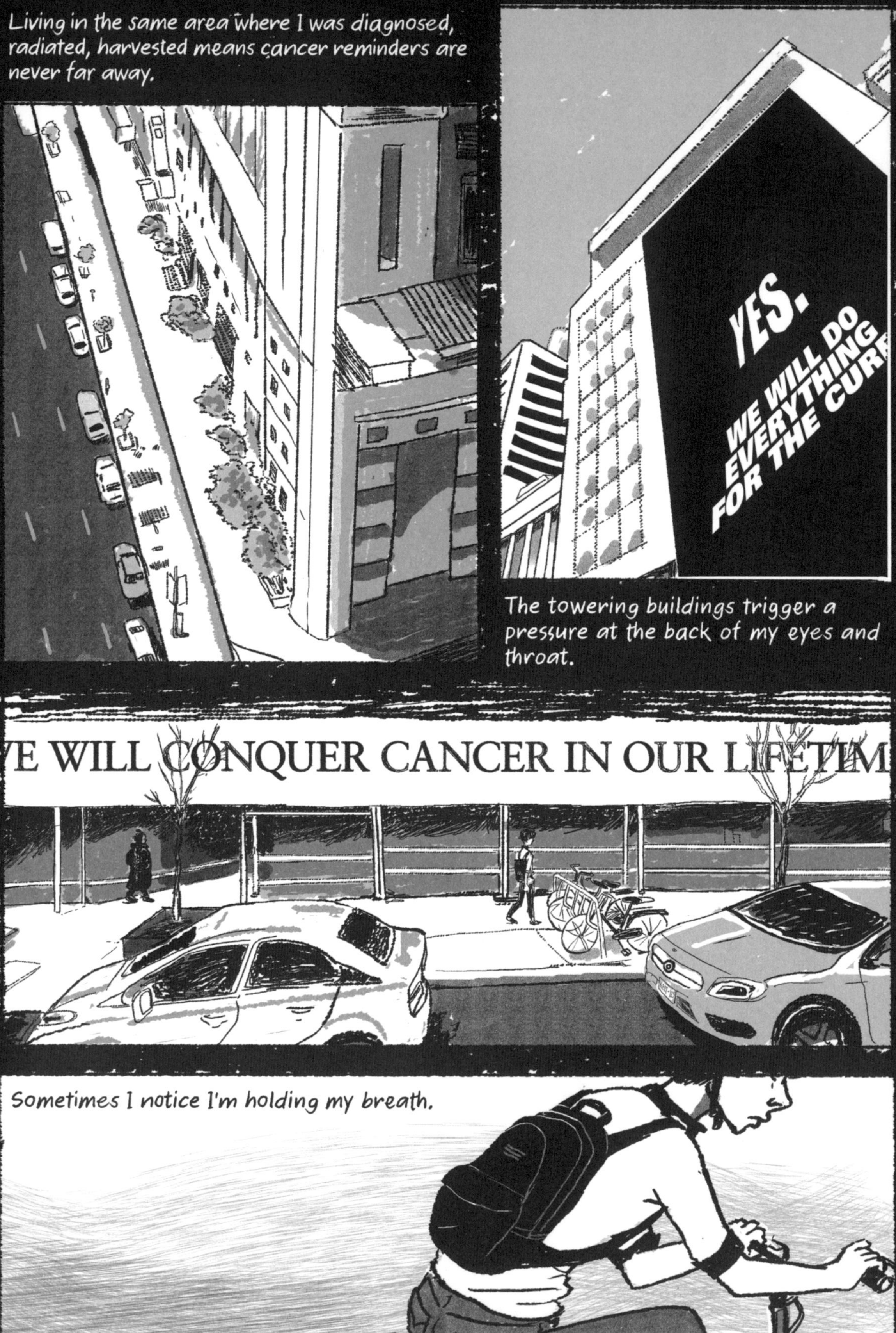
Living in the same area where I was diagnosed, radiated, harvested means cancer reminders are never far away.
YES.
WE WILL DO EVERYTHING FOR THE CUR
The towering buildings trigger a pressure at the back of my eyes and throat.
E WILL CONQUER CANCER IN OUR LIFETIM
Sometimes I notice I'm holding my breath.

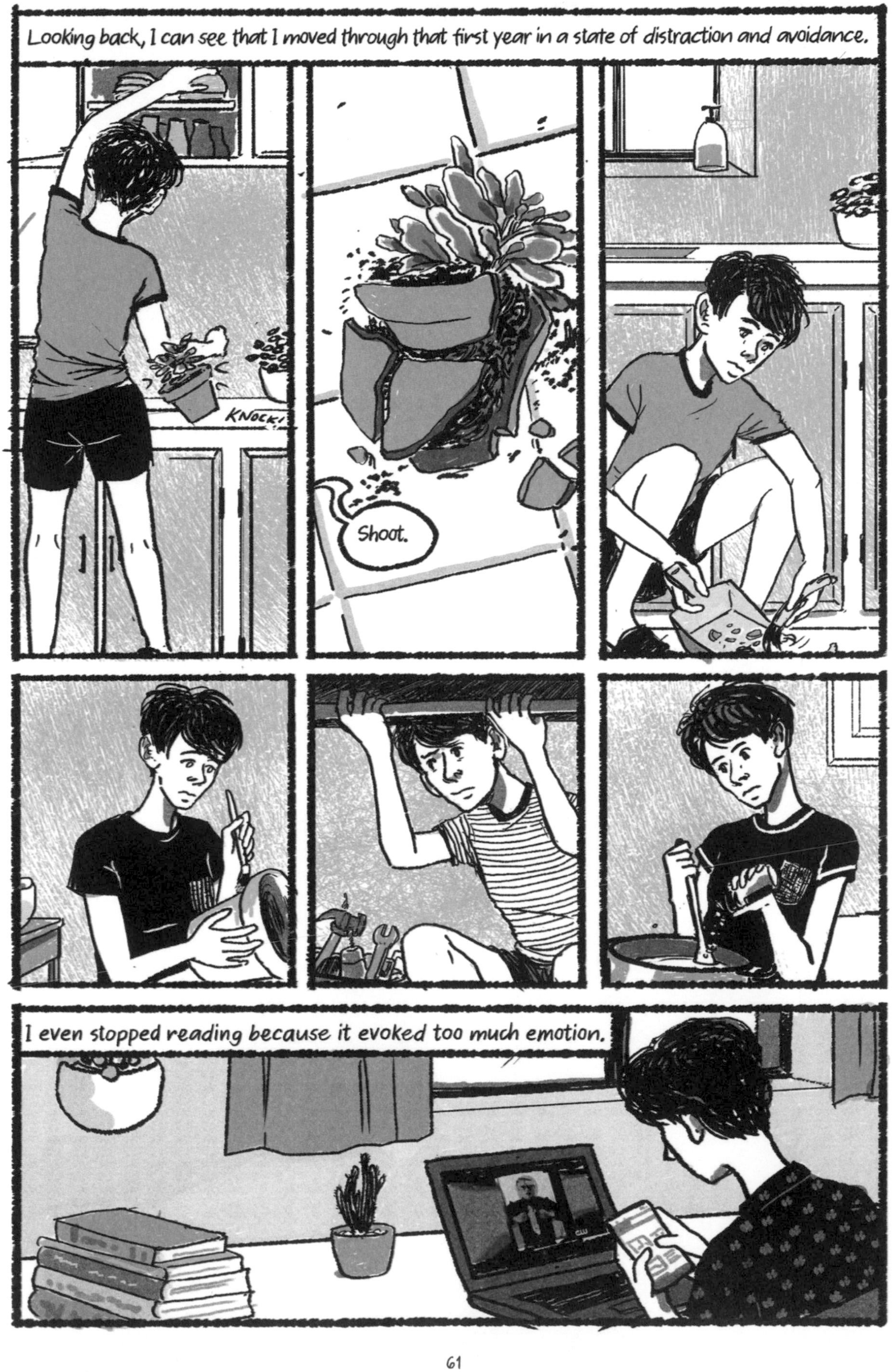
Looking back, I can see that I moved through that first year in a state of distraction and avoidance.
KNOCK!
Shoot.
I even stopped reading because it evoked too much emotion.

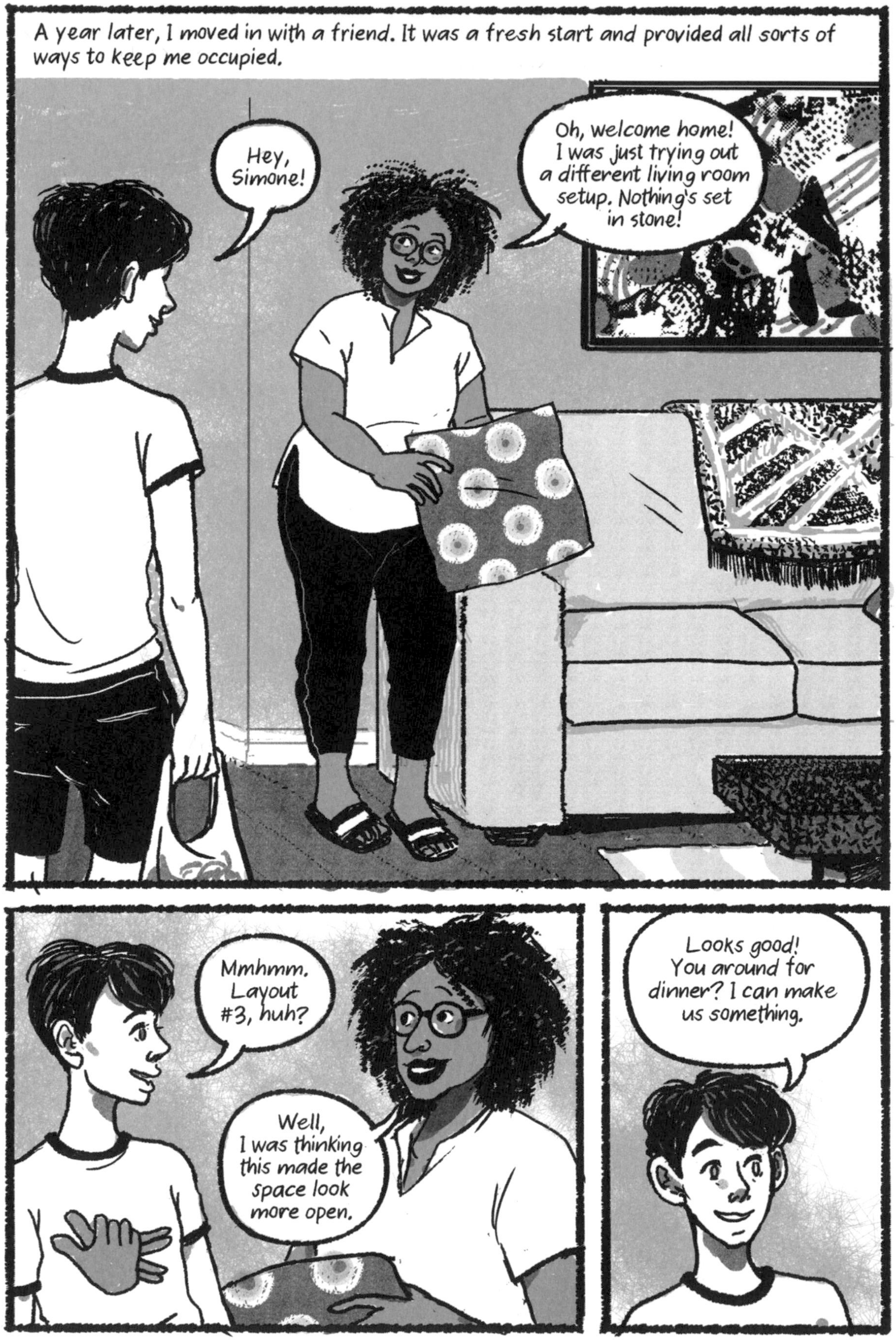
A year later, I moved in with a friend. It was a fresh start and provided all sorts of ways to keep me occupied.
Hey, Simone!
Oh, welcome home! I was just trying out a different living room setup. Nothing's set in stone!
Mmhmm. Layout #3, huh?
Well, I was thinking this made the space look more open.
Looks good! You around for dinner? I can make us something.

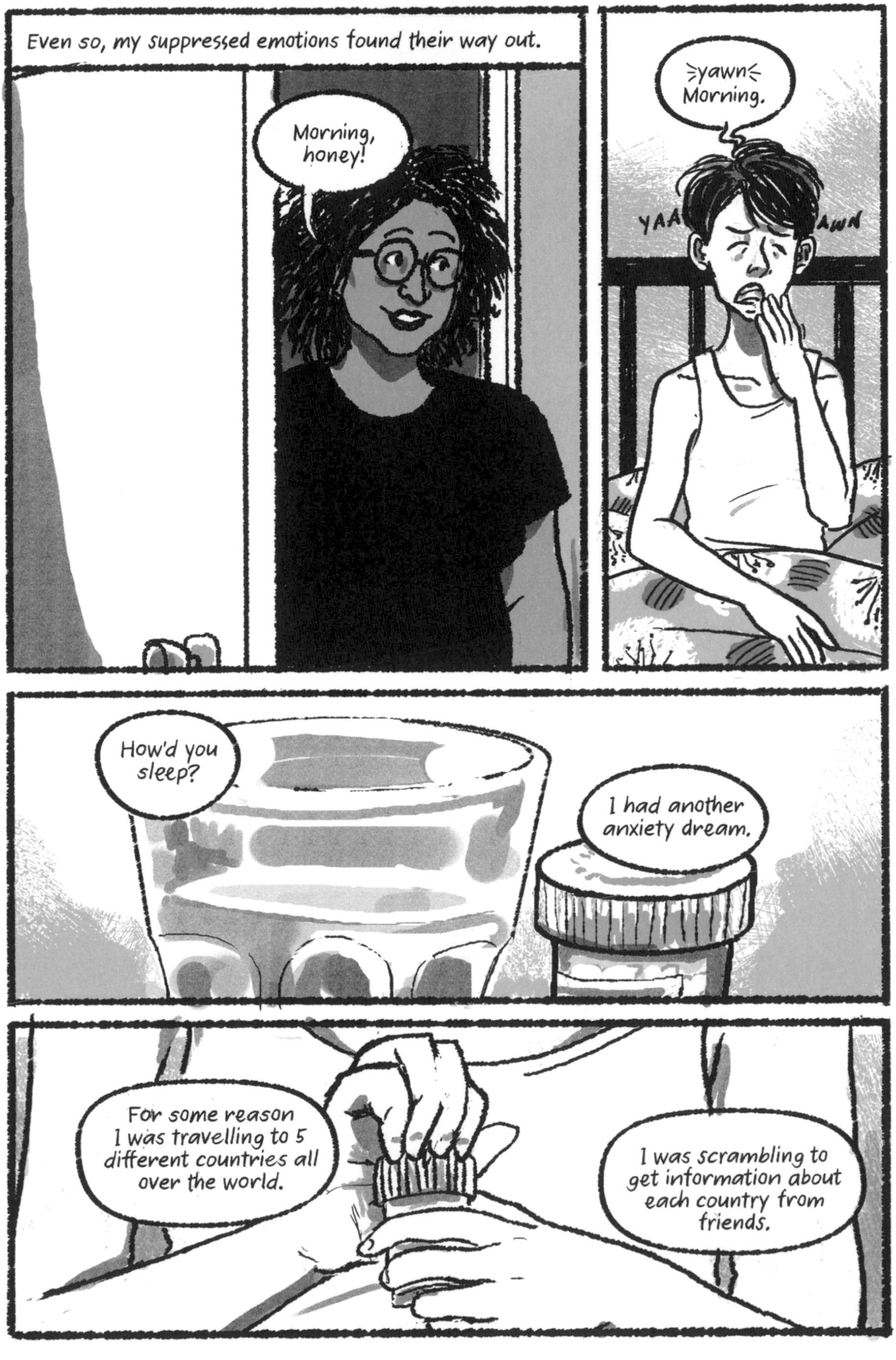
Even so, my suppressed emotions found their way out.
Morning, honey!
yawn Morning.
YAAAWN
How'd you sleep?
I had another anxiety dream.
For some reason I was travelling to 5 different countries all over the world.
I was scrambling to get information about each country from friends.

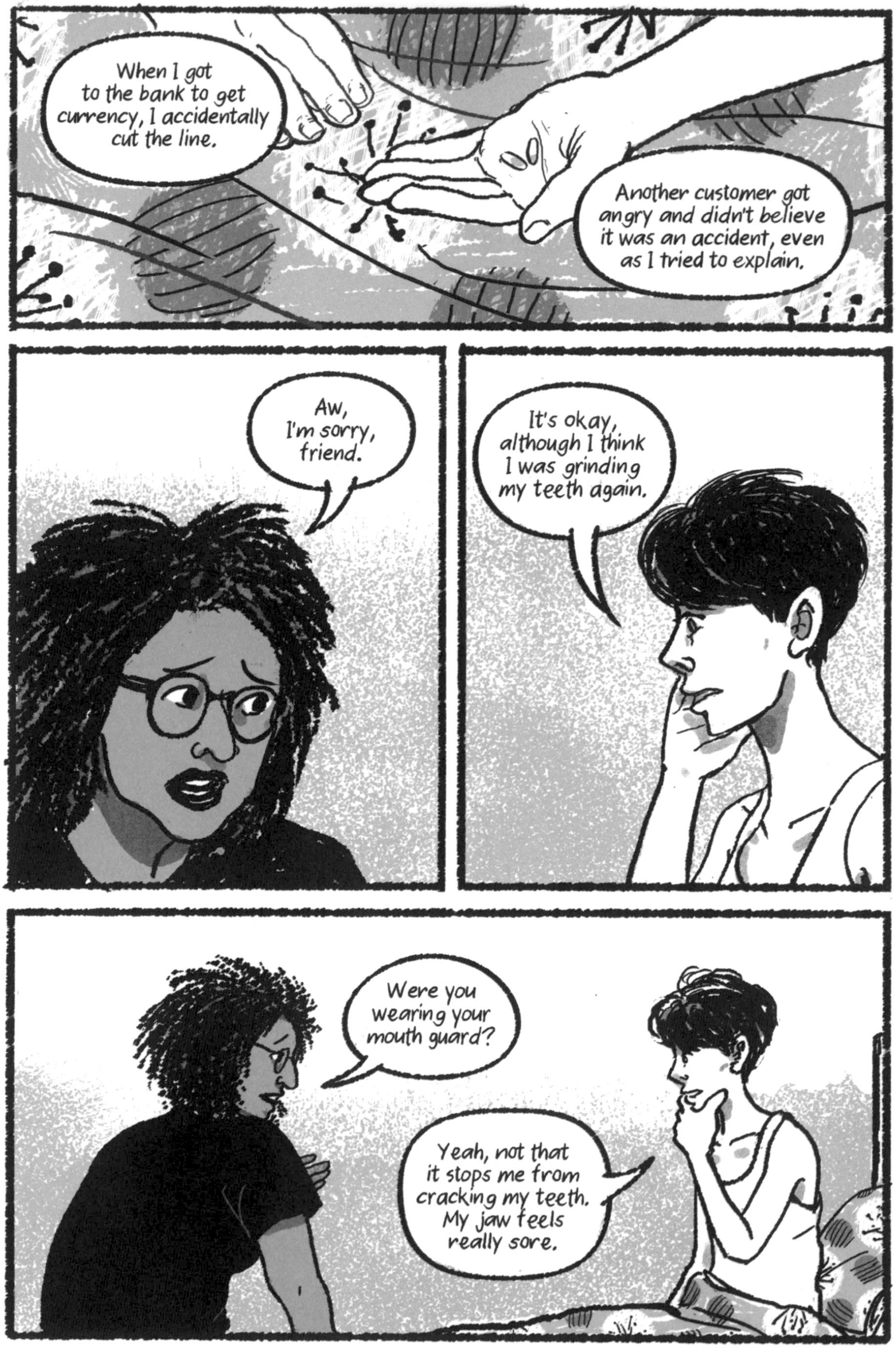
When I got to the bank to get currency, I accidentally cut the line.
Another customer got angry and didn't believe it was an accident, even as I tried to explain.
Aw, I'm sorry, friend.
It's okay, although I think I was grinding my teeth again.
Were you wearing your mouth guard?
Yeah, not that it stops me from cracking my teeth. My jaw feels really sore.

I distinctly recall my last radiation session. Having gotten through surgery, egg harvesting and radiation, it was as if I could suddenly allow myself a little release.

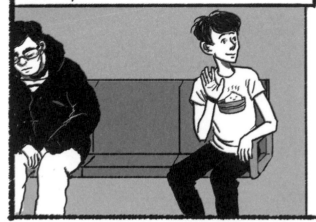

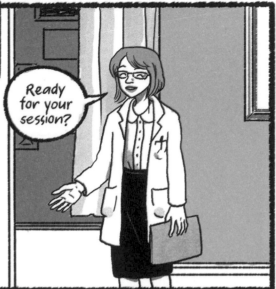

Ready for your session?

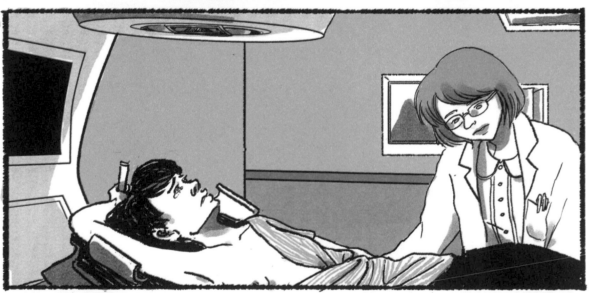

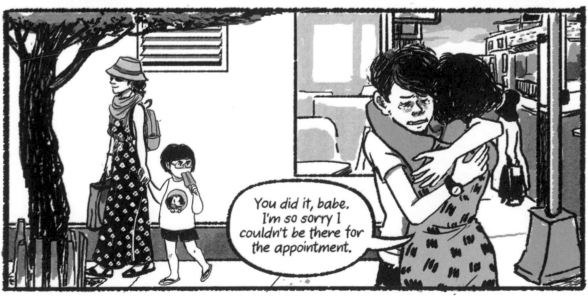

You did it, babe. I'm so sorry I couldn't be there for the appointment.

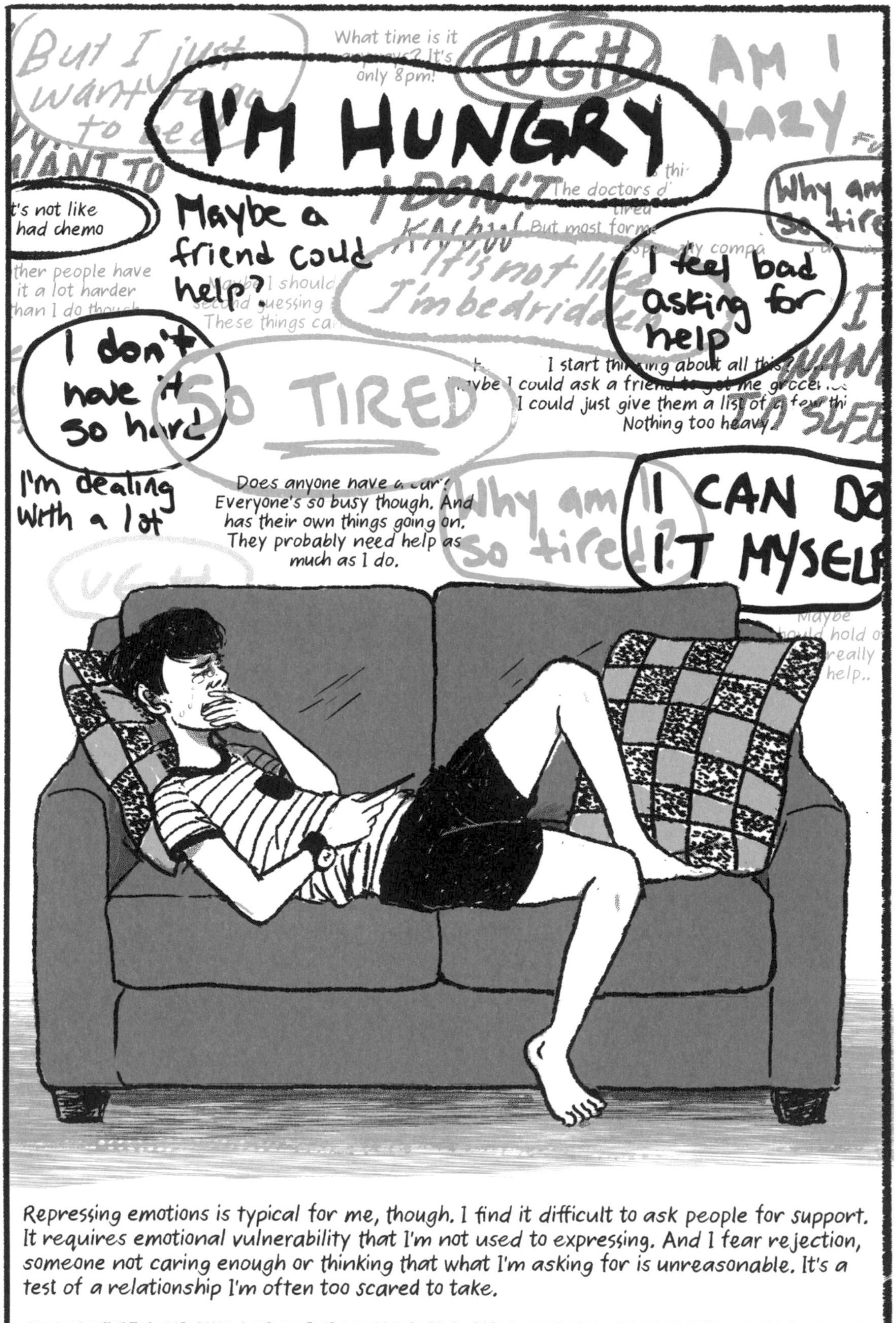
But I just want to go to bed
What time is it anyways? It's only 8pm!
UGH
AM I LAZY
I'M HUNGRY
I DON'T KNOW
Maybe a friend could help?
I feel bad asking for help
It's not like I'm bedridden
Other people have it a lot harder than I do though
These things can
I don't have it so hard
SO TIRED
I start thinking about all this
maybe I could ask a friend to get me groceries
I could just give them a list of a few things
Nothing too heavy.
I'm dealing with a lot
Does anyone have a car?
Everyone's so busy though. And has their own things going on. They probably need help as much as I do.
Why am I so tired?
I CAN DO IT MYSELF
Repressing emotions is typical for me, though. I find it difficult to ask people for support. It requires emotional vulnerability that I'm not used to expressing. And I fear rejection, someone not caring enough or thinking that what I'm asking for is unreasonable. It's a test of a relationship I'm often too scared to take.

It probably doesn't help that I tie my masculinity—and, really, my value—to being able to provide for others. Whether it's running errands, baking or offering emotional support, I tend to focus on my output as the key way I affirm my butchness, dykeness, whatever you want to call it. This isn't sustainable post-cancer.

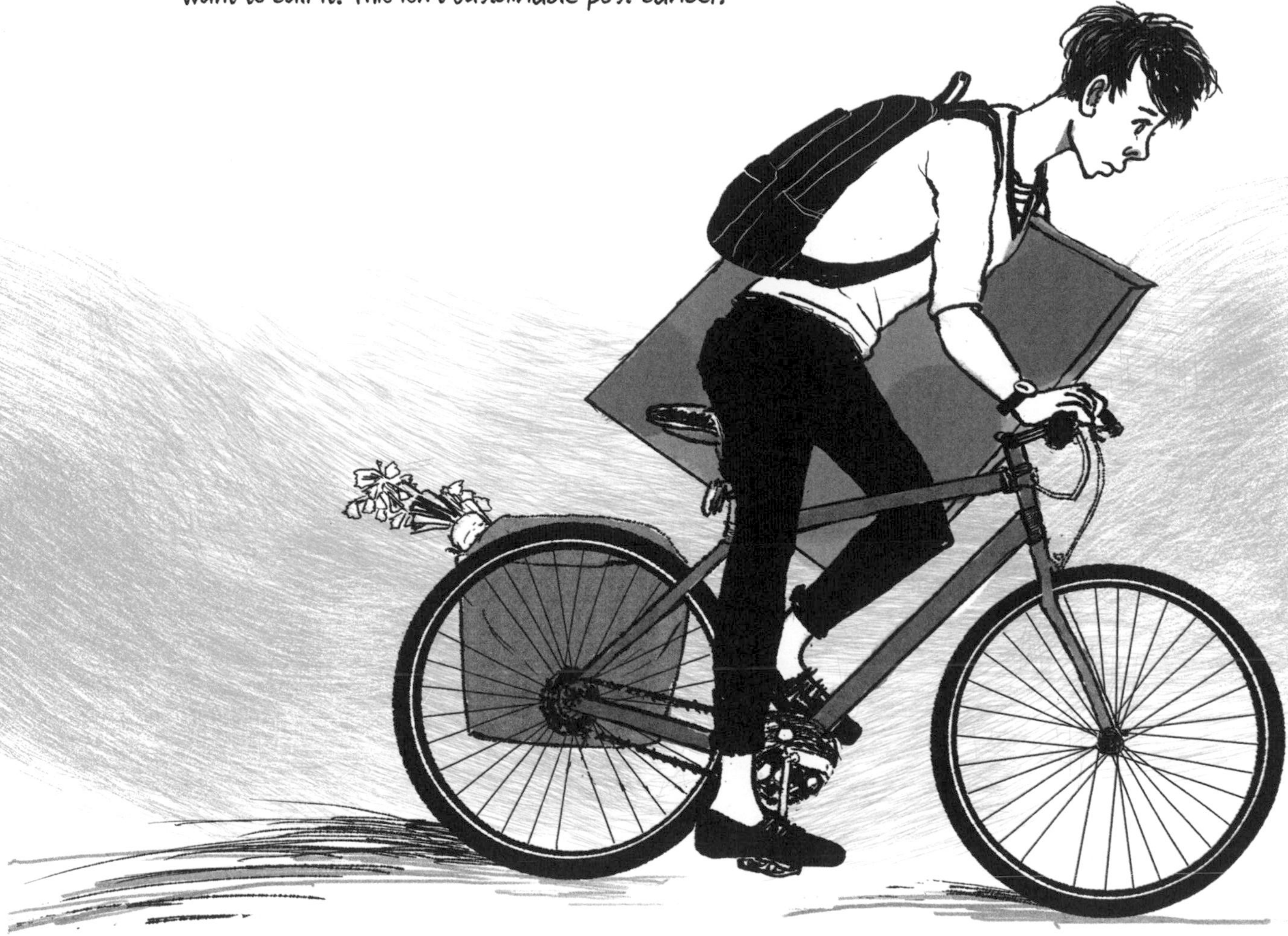

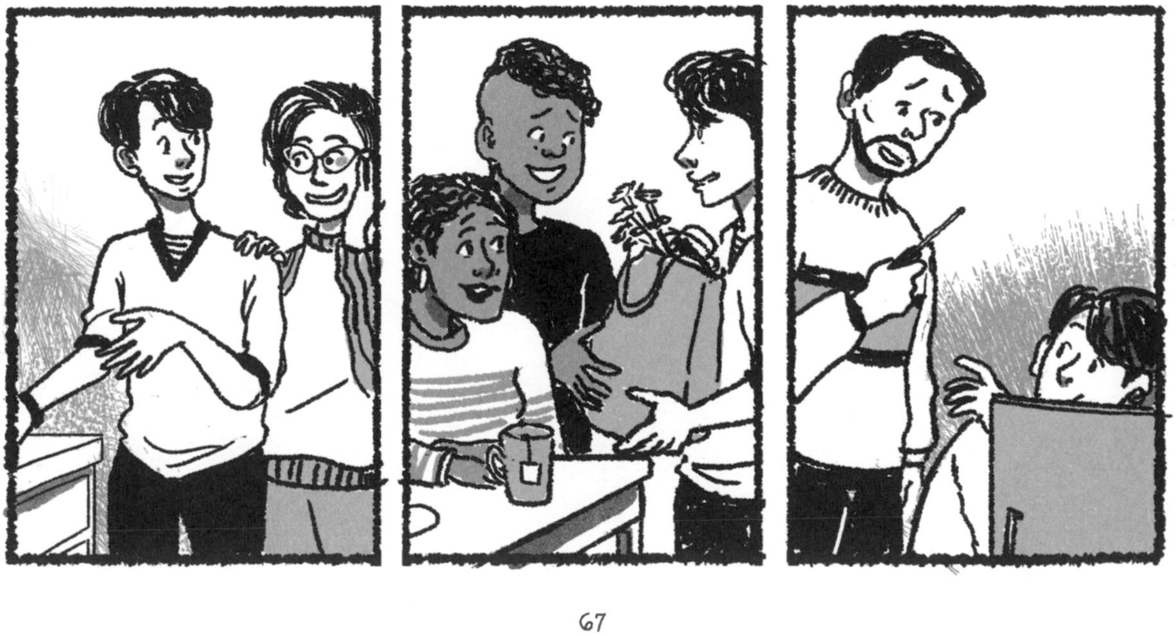

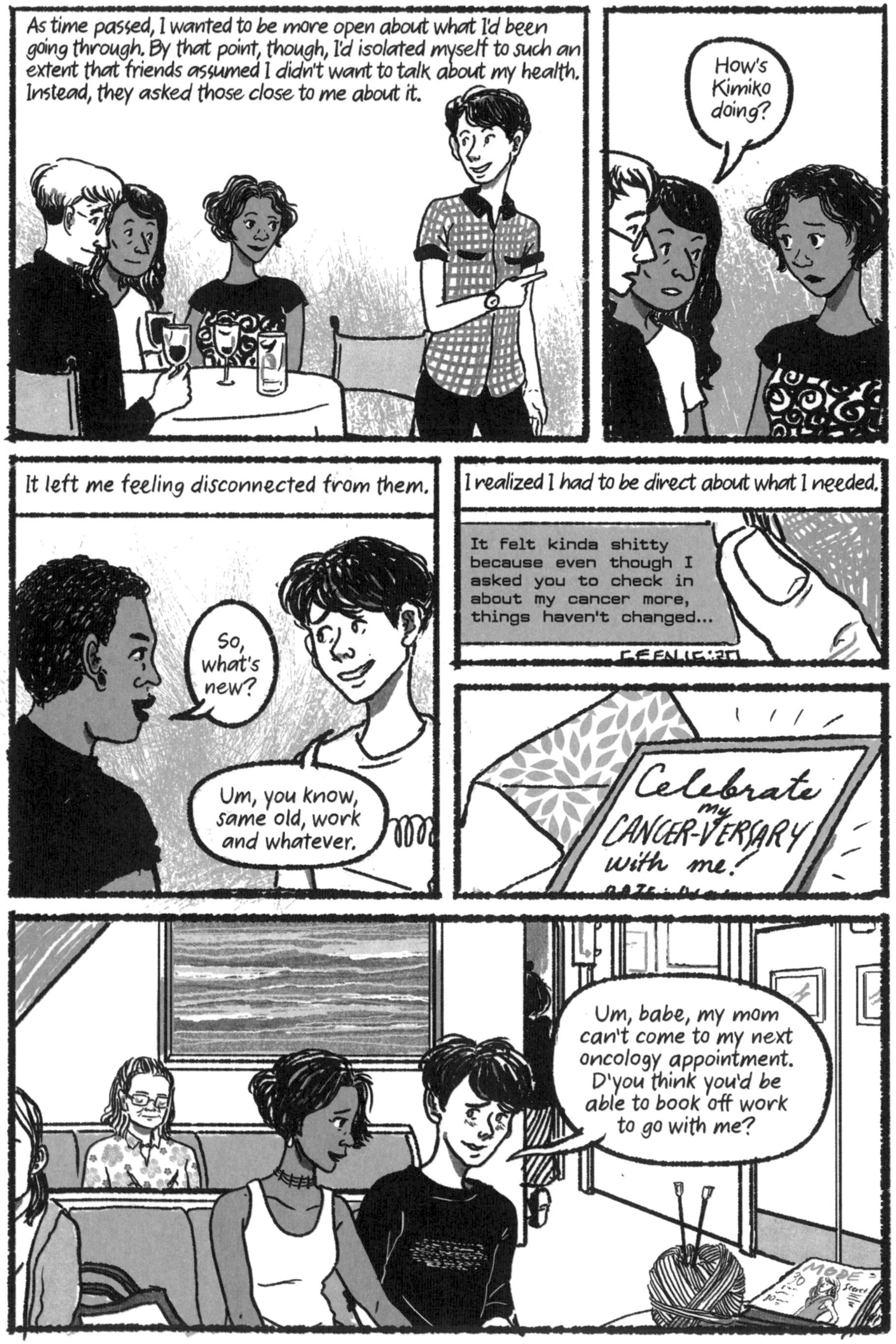
As time passed, I wanted to be more open about what I'd been going through. By that point, though, I'd isolated myself to such an extent that friends assumed I didn't want to talk about my health. Instead, they asked those close to me about it.
How's Kimiko doing?
It left me feeling disconnected from them.
So, what's new?
Um, you know, same old, work and whatever.
I realized I had to be direct about what I needed.
It felt kinda shitty because even though I asked you to check in about my cancer more, things haven't changed...
Celebrate my CANCER-VERSARY with me!
Um, babe, my mom can't come to my next oncology appointment. D'you think you'd be able to book off work to go with me?

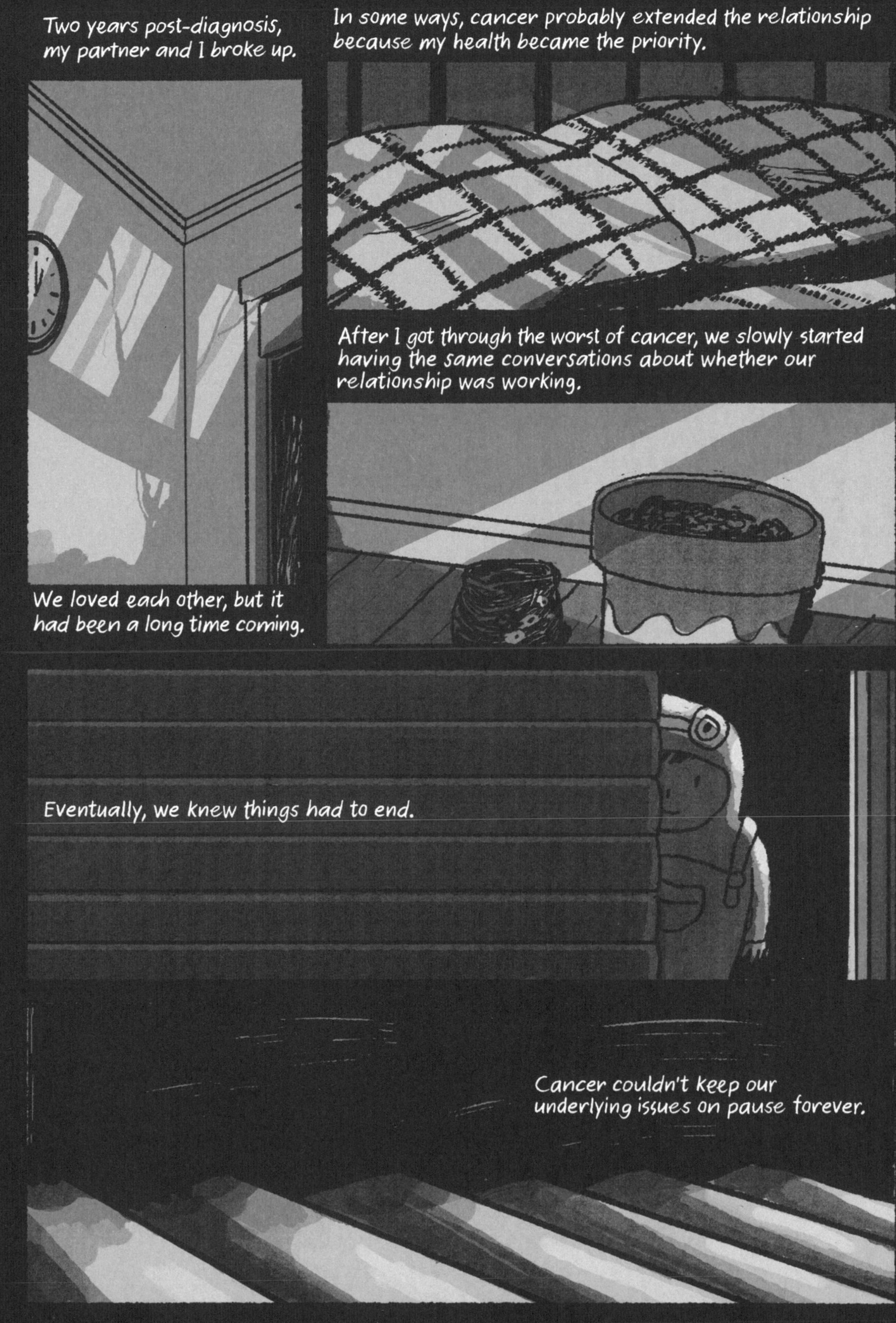

Two years post-diagnosis, my partner and I broke up.

In some ways, cancer probably extended the relationship because my health became the priority.

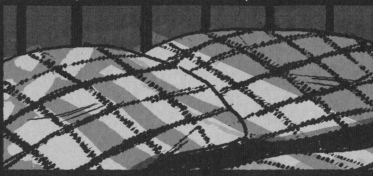

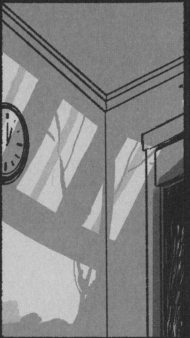

After I got through the worst of cancer, we slowly started having the same conversations about whether our relationship was working.

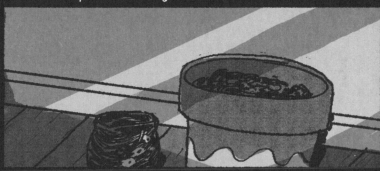

We loved each other, but it had been a long time coming.

Eventually, we knew things had to end.

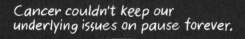

Cancer couldn't keep our underlying issues on pause forever.

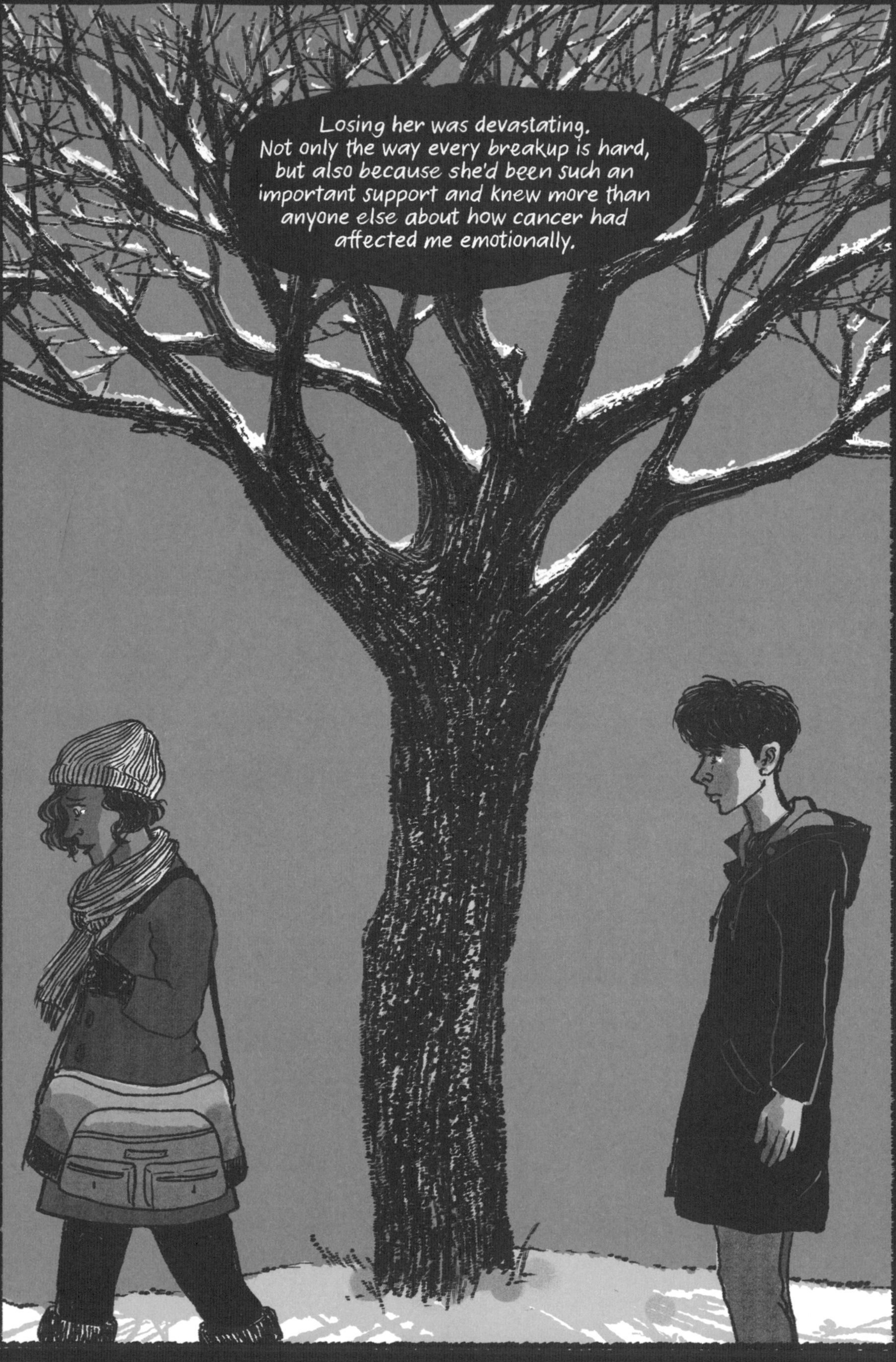
Losing her was devastating. Not only the way every breakup is hard, but also because she'd been such an important support and knew more than anyone else about how cancer had affected me emotionally.

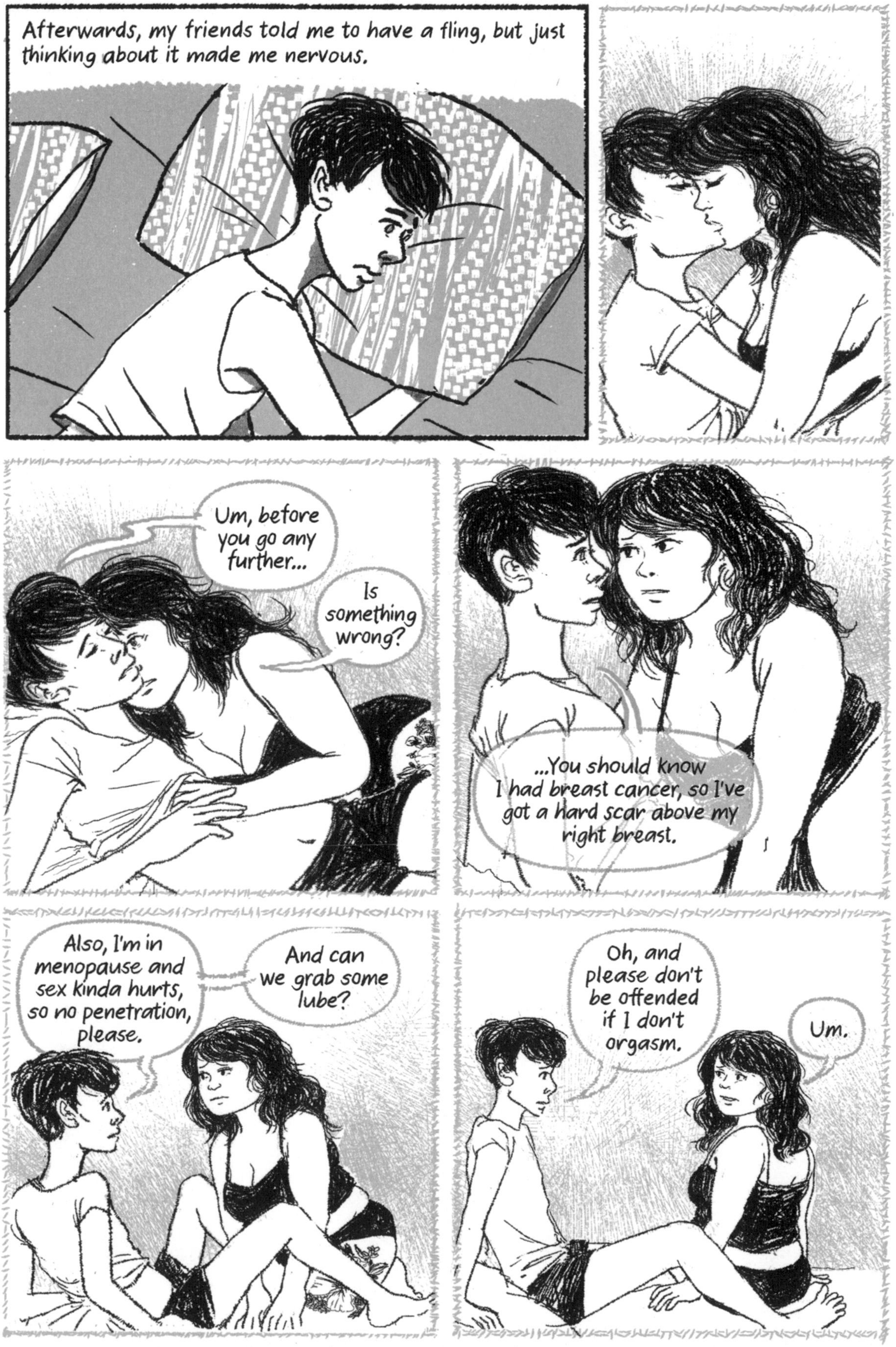
Afterwards, my friends told me to have a fling, but just thinking about it made me nervous.
Um, before you go any further...
Is something wrong?
...You should know I had breast cancer, so I've got a hard scar above my right breast.
Also, I'm in menopause and sex kinda hurts, so no penetration, please.
And can we grab some lube?
Oh, and please don't be offended if I don't orgasm.
Um.

There are a lot of conversations I'm still figuring out how to navigate, like telling a new acquaintance I had cancer. It either falls flat because they don't understand, or it evokes a strong reaction that I have to manage. It's a complicated balance.

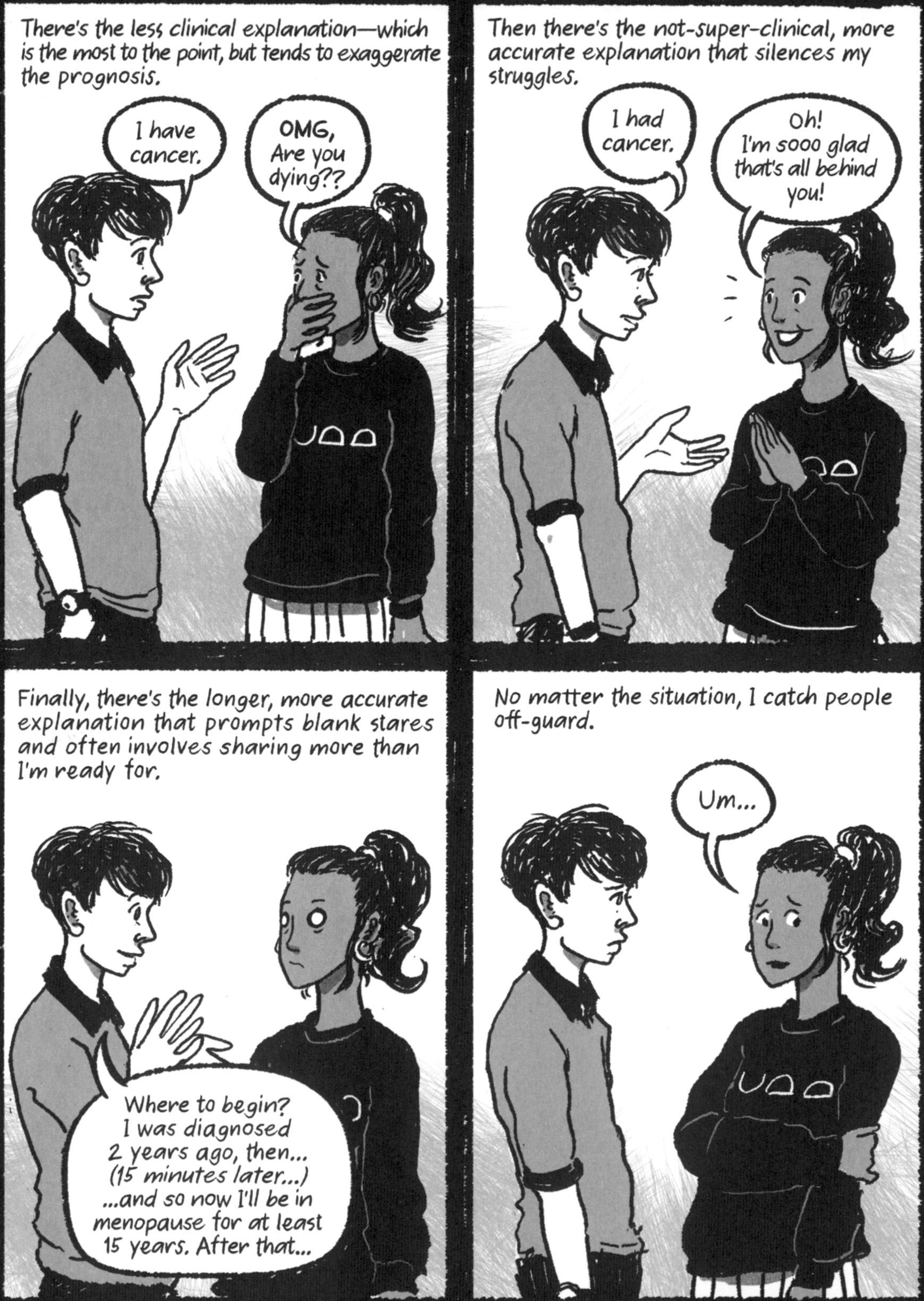
There's the less clinical explanation—which is the most to the point, but tends to exaggerate the prognosis.
I have cancer.
OMG, Are you dying??
Then there's the not-super-clinical, more accurate explanation that silences my struggles.
I had cancer.
Oh! I'm sooo glad that's all behind you!
Finally, there's the longer, more accurate explanation that prompts blank stares and often involves sharing more than I'm ready for.
Where to begin? I was diagnosed 2 years ago, then... (15 minutes later...) ...and so now I'll be in menopause for at least 15 years. After that...
No matter the situation, I catch people off-guard.
Um...

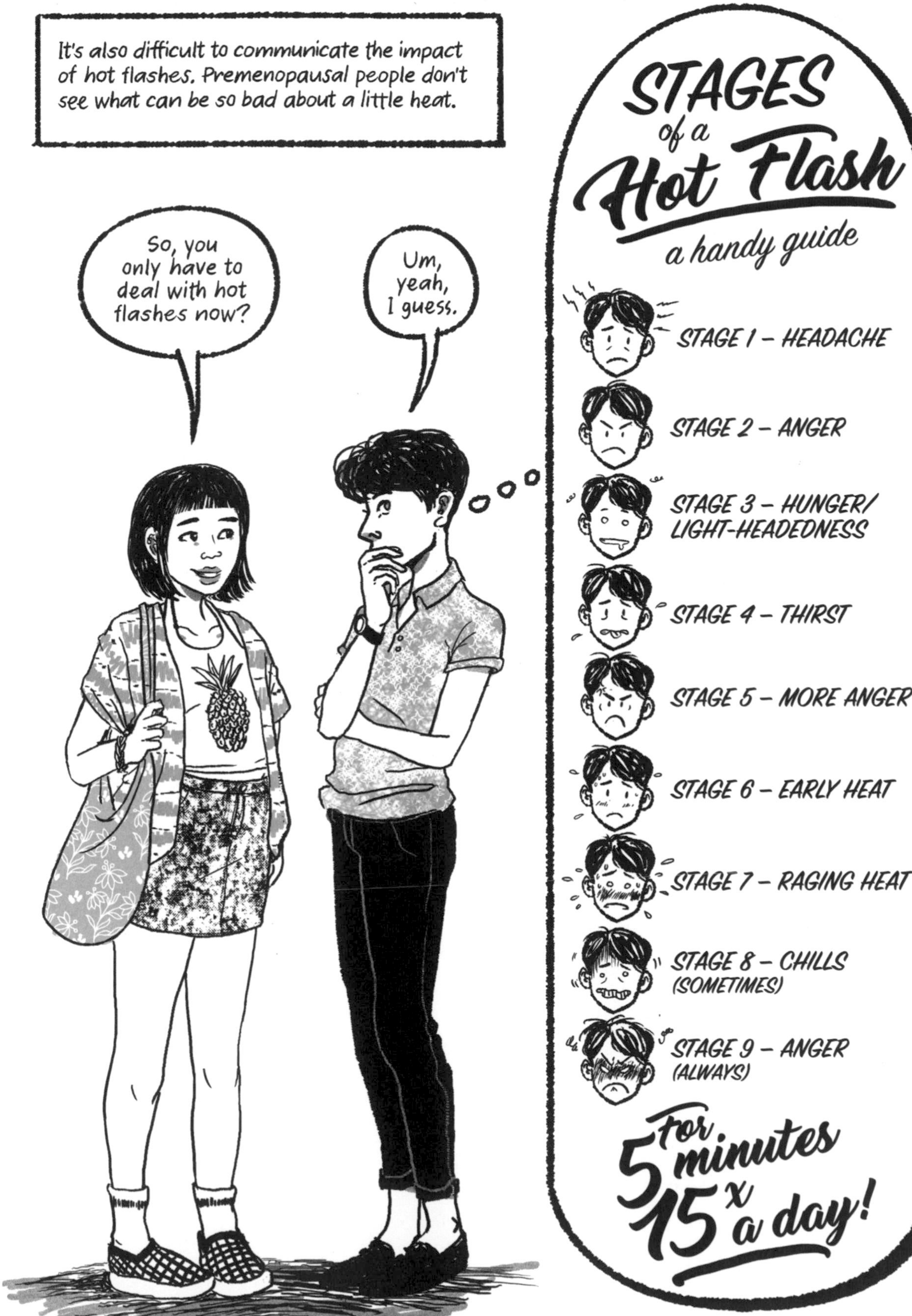
It's also difficult to communicate the impact of hot flashes. Premenopausal people don't see what can be so bad about a little heat.
So, you only have to deal with hot flashes now?
Um, yeah, I guess.
STAGES of a Hot Flash
a handy guide
STAGE 1 – HEADACHE
STAGE 2 – ANGER
STAGE 3 – HUNGER/ LIGHT-HEADEDNESS
STAGE 4 – THIRST
STAGE 5 – MORE ANGER
STAGE 6 – EARLY HEAT
STAGE 7 – RAGING HEAT
STAGE 8 – CHILLS (SOMETIMES)
STAGE 9 – ANGER (ALWAYS)
For 5 minutes 15 x a day!

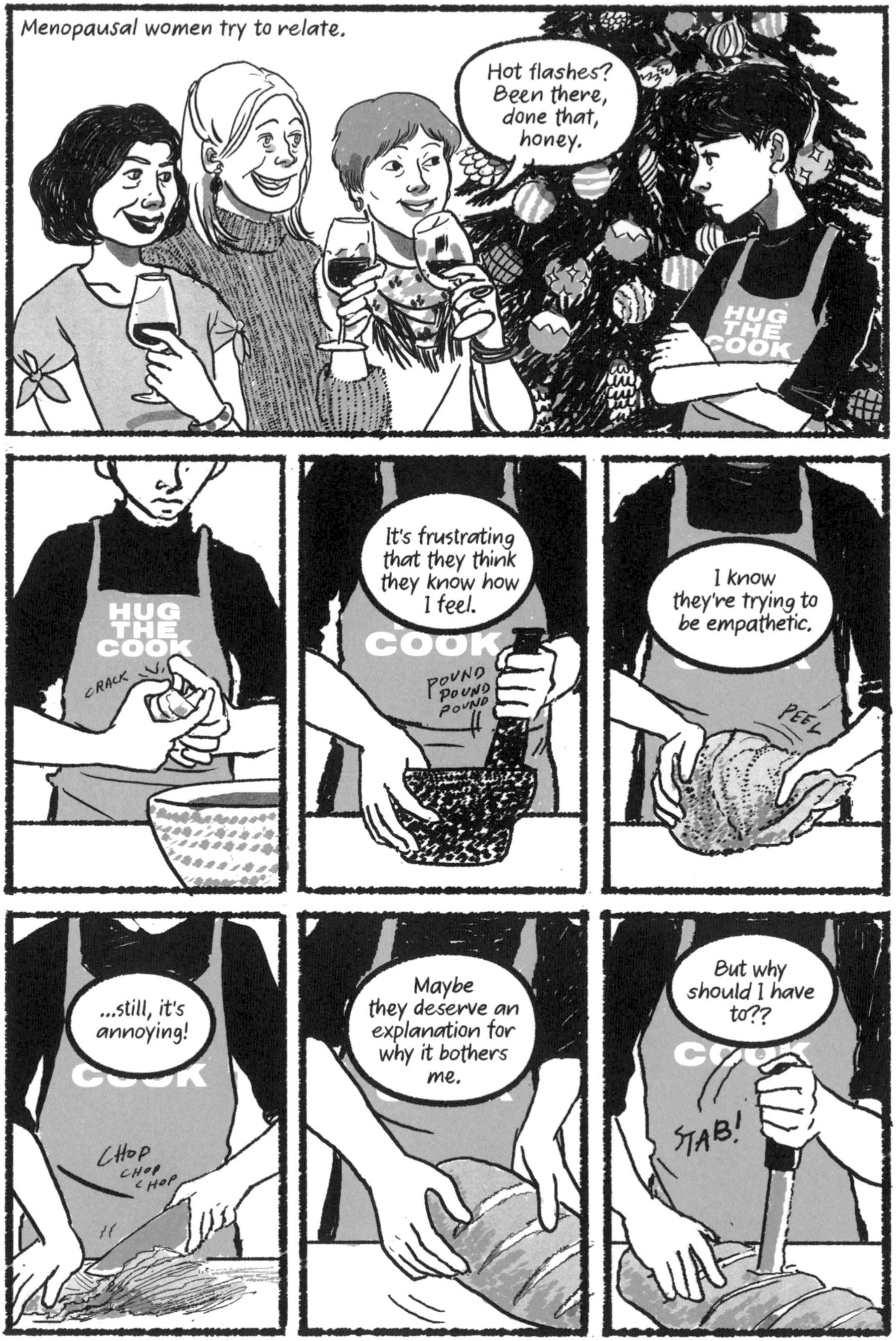
Menopausal women try to relate.
Hot flashes? Been there, done that, honey.
HUG THE COOK
HUG THE COOK
CRACK
It's frustrating that they think they know how I feel.
COOK
POUND POUND POUND
I know they're trying to be empathetic.
PEEL
...still, it's annoying!
COOK
CHOP CHOP CHOP
Maybe they deserve an explanation for why it bothers me.
But why should I have to??
STAB!

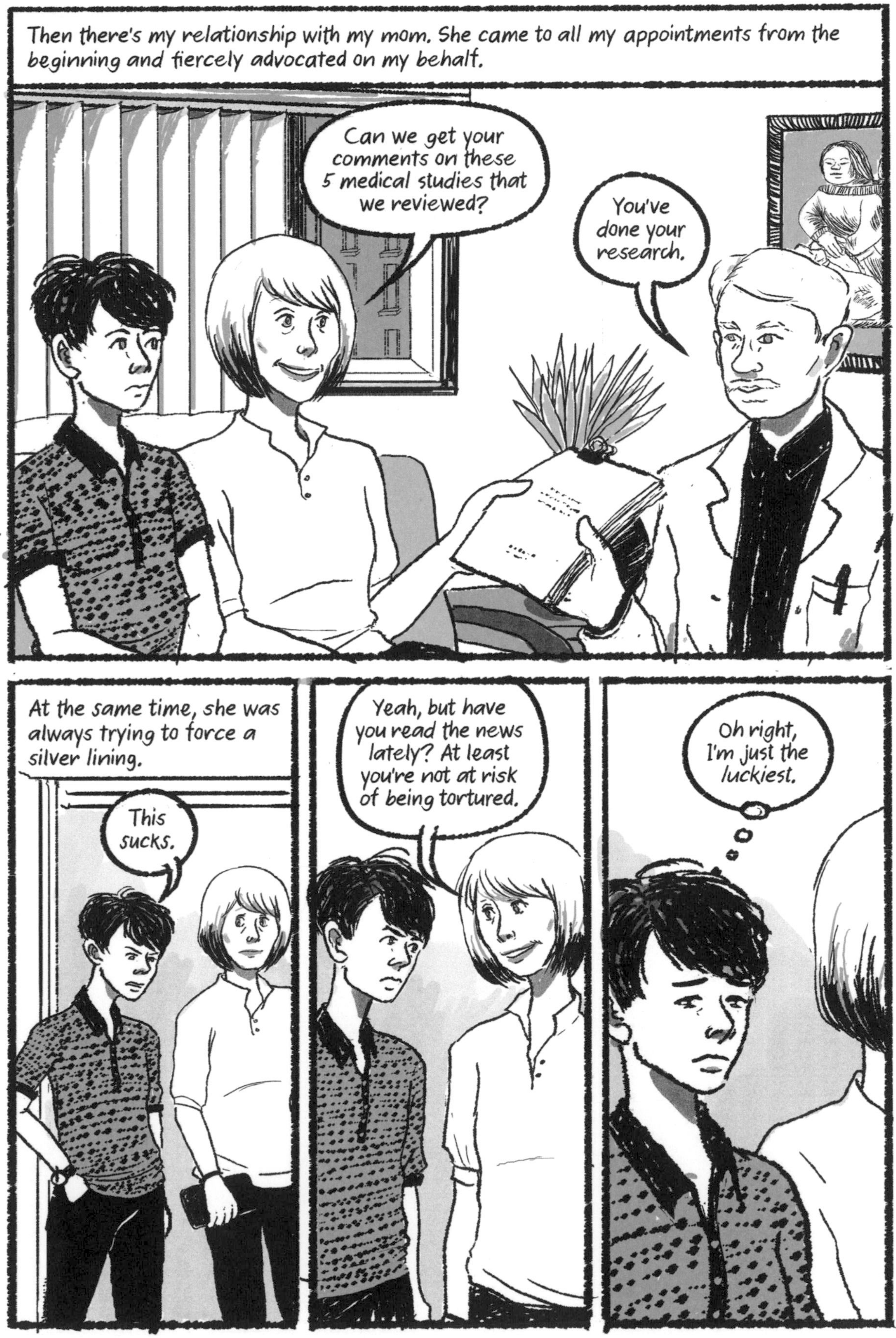
Then there's my relationship with my mom. She came to all my appointments from the beginning and fiercely advocated on my behalf.
Can we get your comments on these 5 medical studies that we reviewed?
You've done your research.
At the same time, she was always trying to force a silver lining.
This sucks.
Yeah, but have you read the news lately? At least you're not at risk of being tortured.
Oh right, I'm just the luckiest.

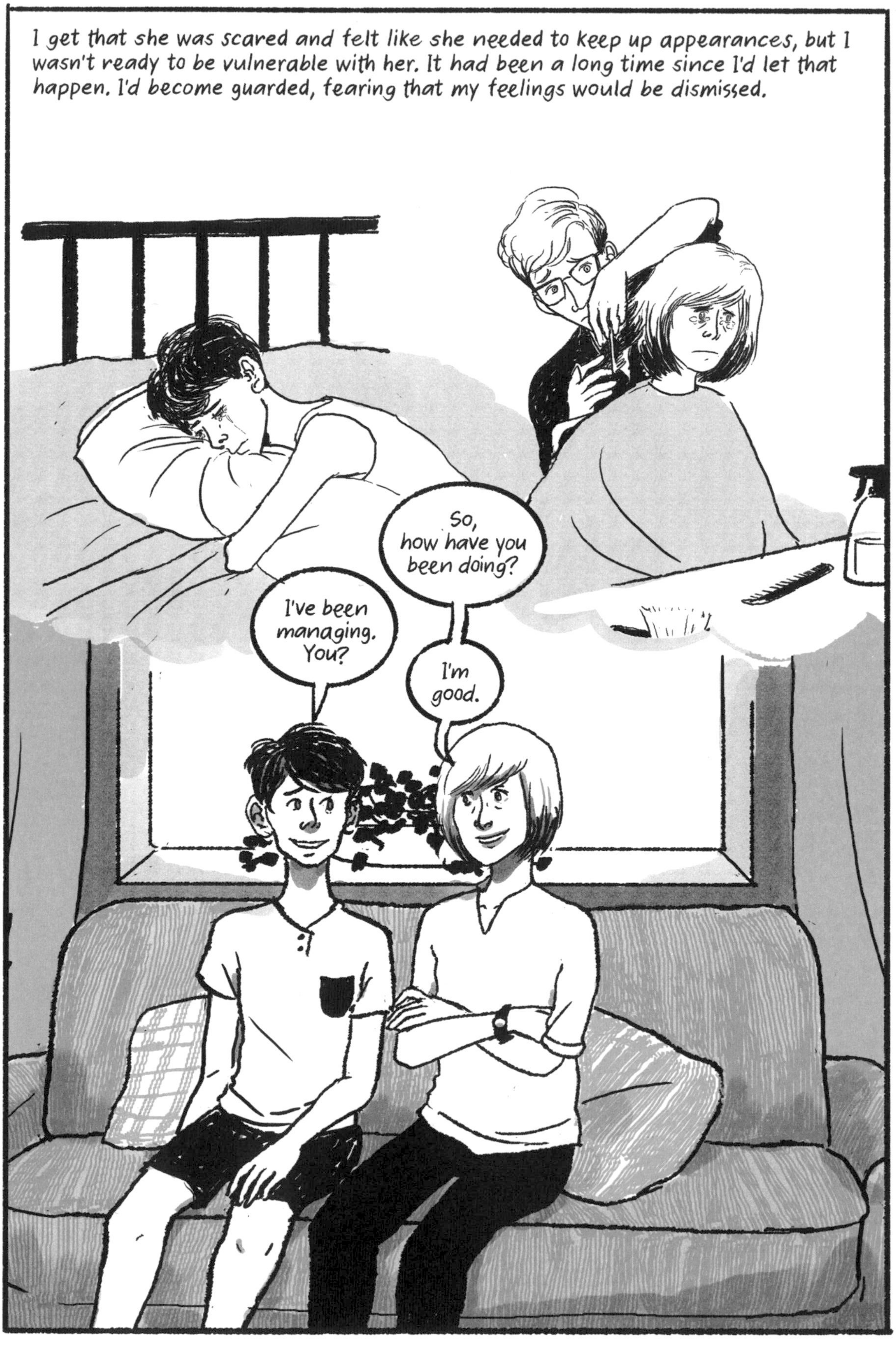
I get that she was scared and felt like she needed to keep up appearances, but I wasn't ready to be vulnerable with her. It had been a long time since I'd let that happen. I'd become guarded, fearing that my feelings would be dismissed.
So, how have you been doing?
I've been managing. You?
I'm good.

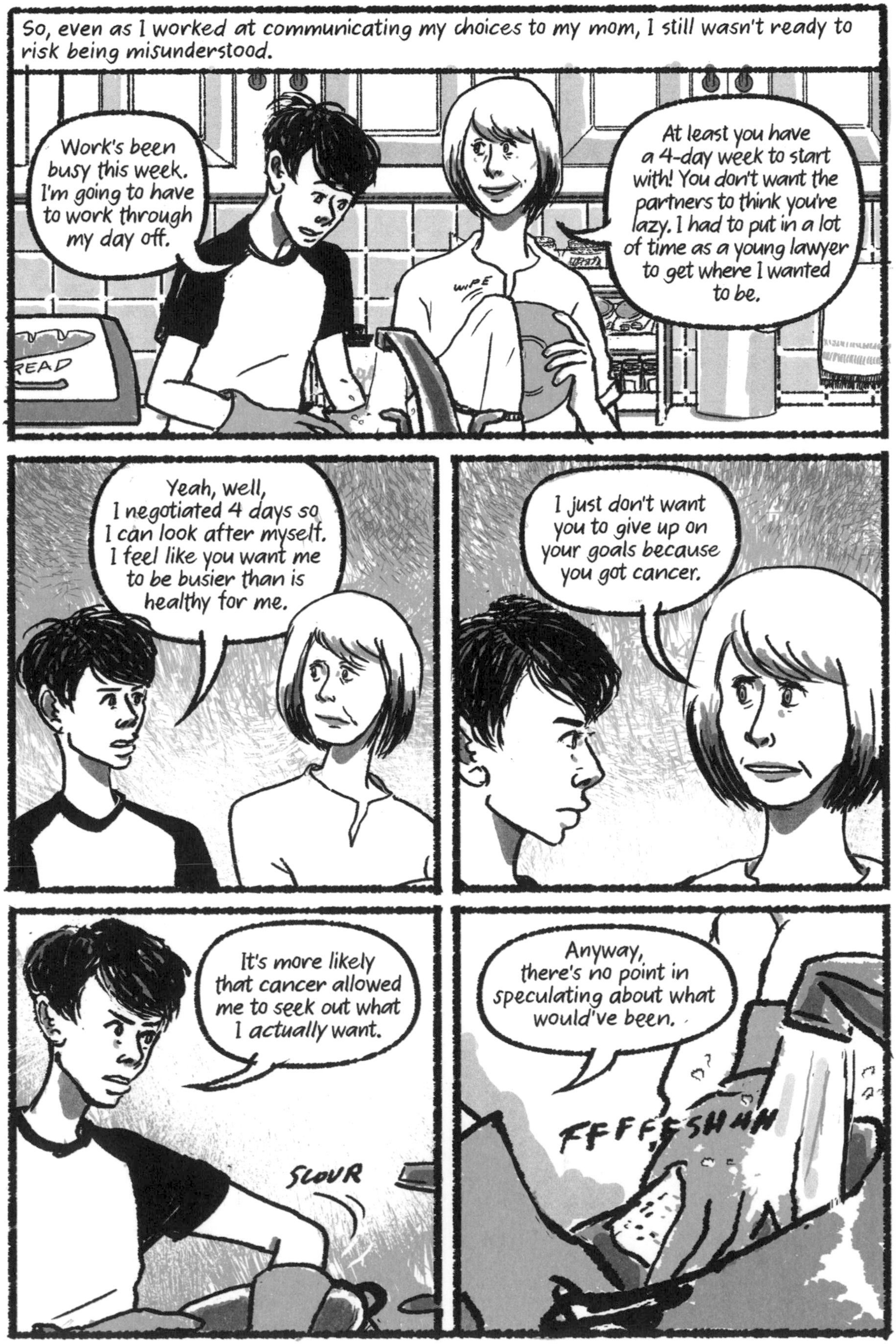
So, even as I worked at communicating my choices to my mom, I still wasn't ready to risk being misunderstood.
Work's been busy this week. I'm going to have to work through my day off.
At least you have a 4-day week to start with! You don't want the partners to think you're lazy. I had to put in a lot of time as a young lawyer to get where I wanted to be.
WIPE
READ
Yeah, well, I negotiated 4 days so I can look after myself. I feel like you want me to be busier than is healthy for me.
I just don't want you to give up on your goals because you got cancer.
It's more likely that cancer allowed me to seek out what I actually want.
SCOUR
Anyway, there's no point in speculating about what would've been.
FFFFFSHHH

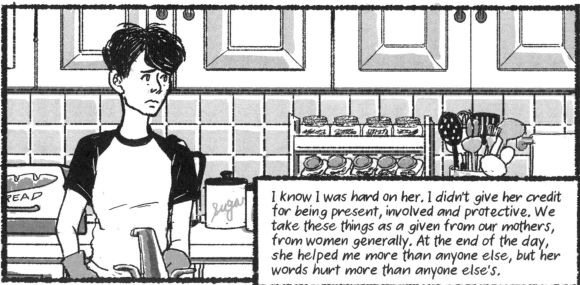

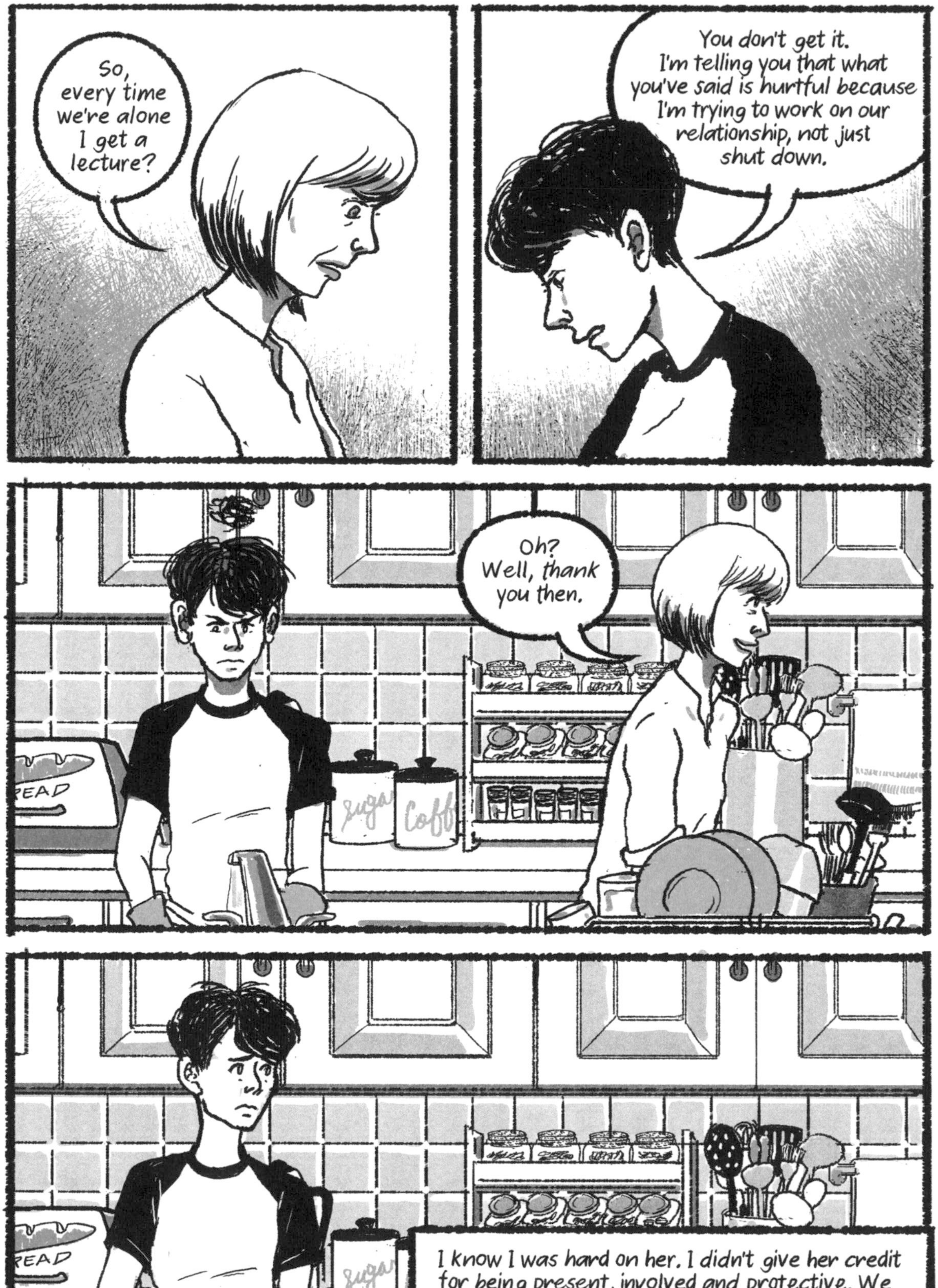
So, every time we're alone I get a lecture?
You don't get it. I'm telling you that what you've said is hurtful because I'm trying to work on our relationship, not just shut down.
Oh? Well, thank you then.
I know I was hard on her. I didn't give her credit for being present, involved and protective. We take these things as a given from our mothers, from women generally. At the end of the day, she helped me more than anyone else, but her words hurt more than anyone else's.

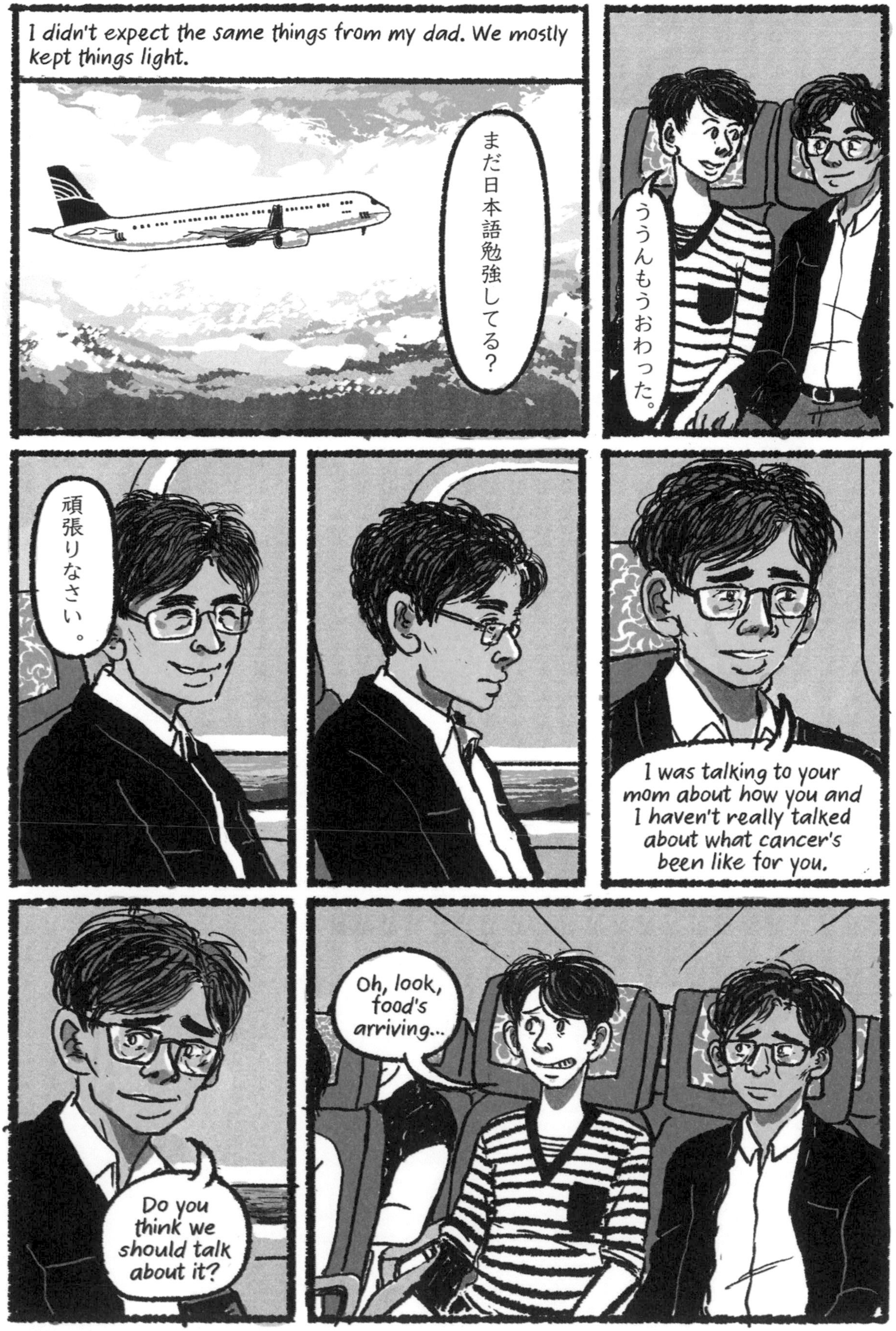
I didn't expect the same things from my dad. We mostly kept things light.
まだ日本語勉強してる？
ううんもうおわった。
頑張りなさい。
I was talking to your mom about how you and I haven't really talked about what cancer's been like for you.
Do you think we should talk about it?
Oh, look, food's arriving...

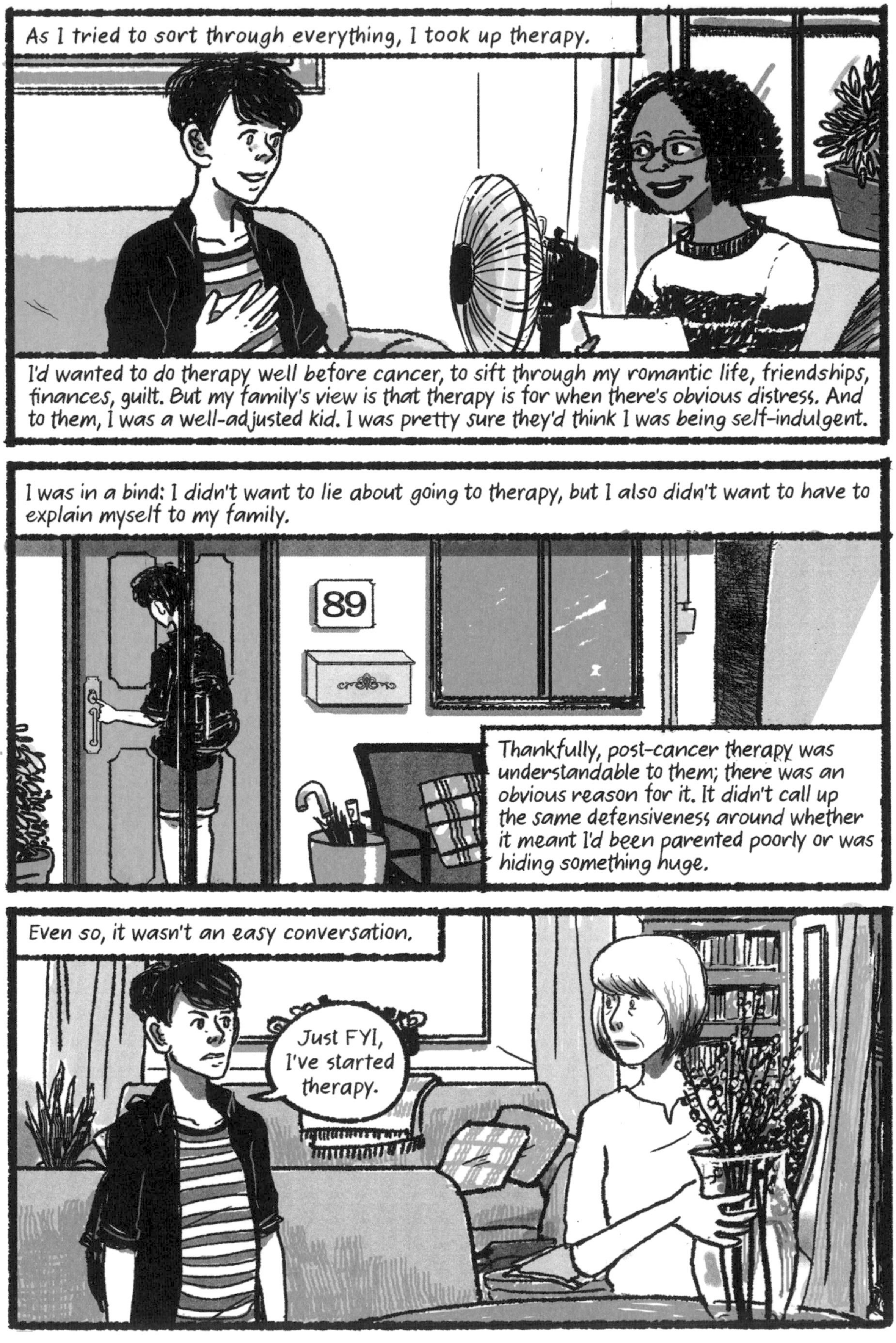
As I tried to sort through everything, I took up therapy.
I'd wanted to do therapy well before cancer, to sift through my romantic life, friendships, finances, guilt. But my family's view is that therapy is for when there's obvious distress. And to them, I was a well-adjusted kid. I was pretty sure they'd think I was being self-indulgent.
I was in a bind: I didn't want to lie about going to therapy, but I also didn't want to have to explain myself to my family.
89
Thankfully, post-cancer therapy was understandable to them; there was an obvious reason for it. It didn't call up the same defensiveness around whether it meant I'd been parented poorly or was hiding something huge.
Even so, it wasn't an easy conversation.
Just FYI, I've started therapy.

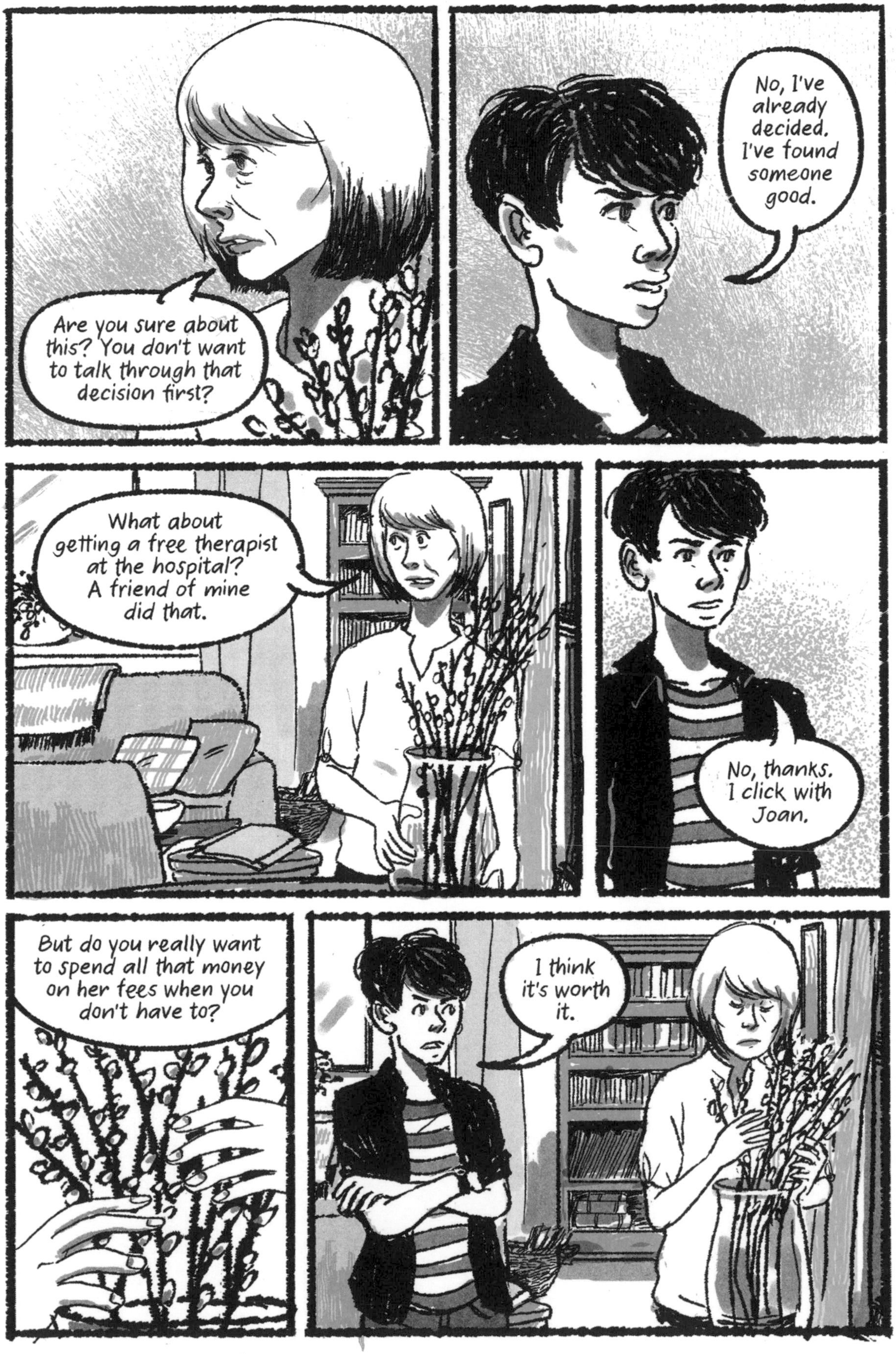
Are you sure about this? You don't want to talk through that decision first?
No, I've already decided. I've found someone good.
What about getting a free therapist at the hospital? A friend of mine did that.
No, thanks. I click with Joan.
But do you really want to spend all that money on her fees when you don't have to?
I think it's worth it.

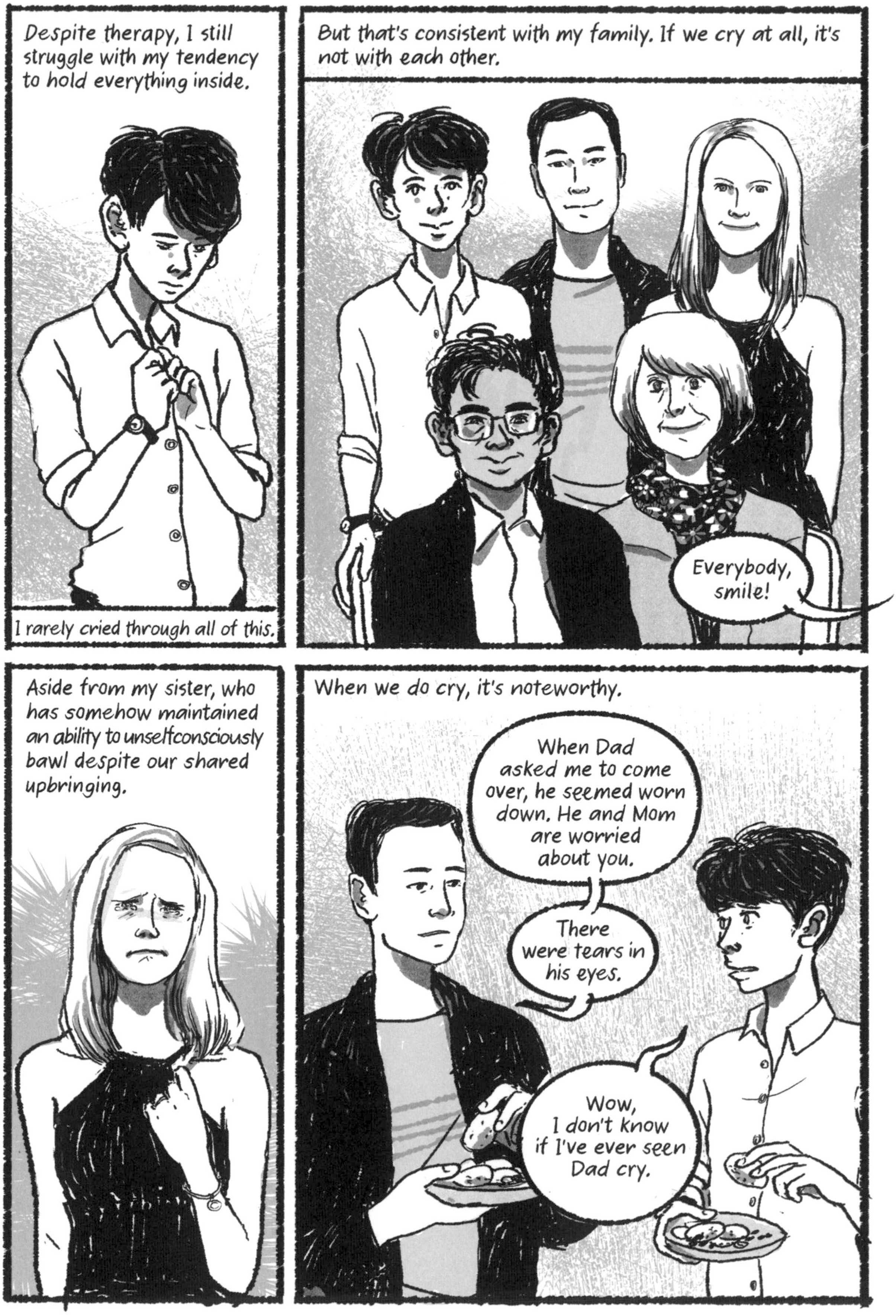
Despite therapy, I still struggle with my tendency to hold everything inside.
I rarely cried through all of this.
But that's consistent with my family. If we cry at all, it's not with each other.
Everybody, smile!
Aside from my sister, who has somehow maintained an ability to unselfconsciously bawl despite our shared upbringing.
When we do cry, it's noteworthy.
When Dad asked me to come over, he seemed worn down. He and Mom are worried about you.
There were tears in his eyes.
Wow, I don't know if I've ever seen Dad cry.

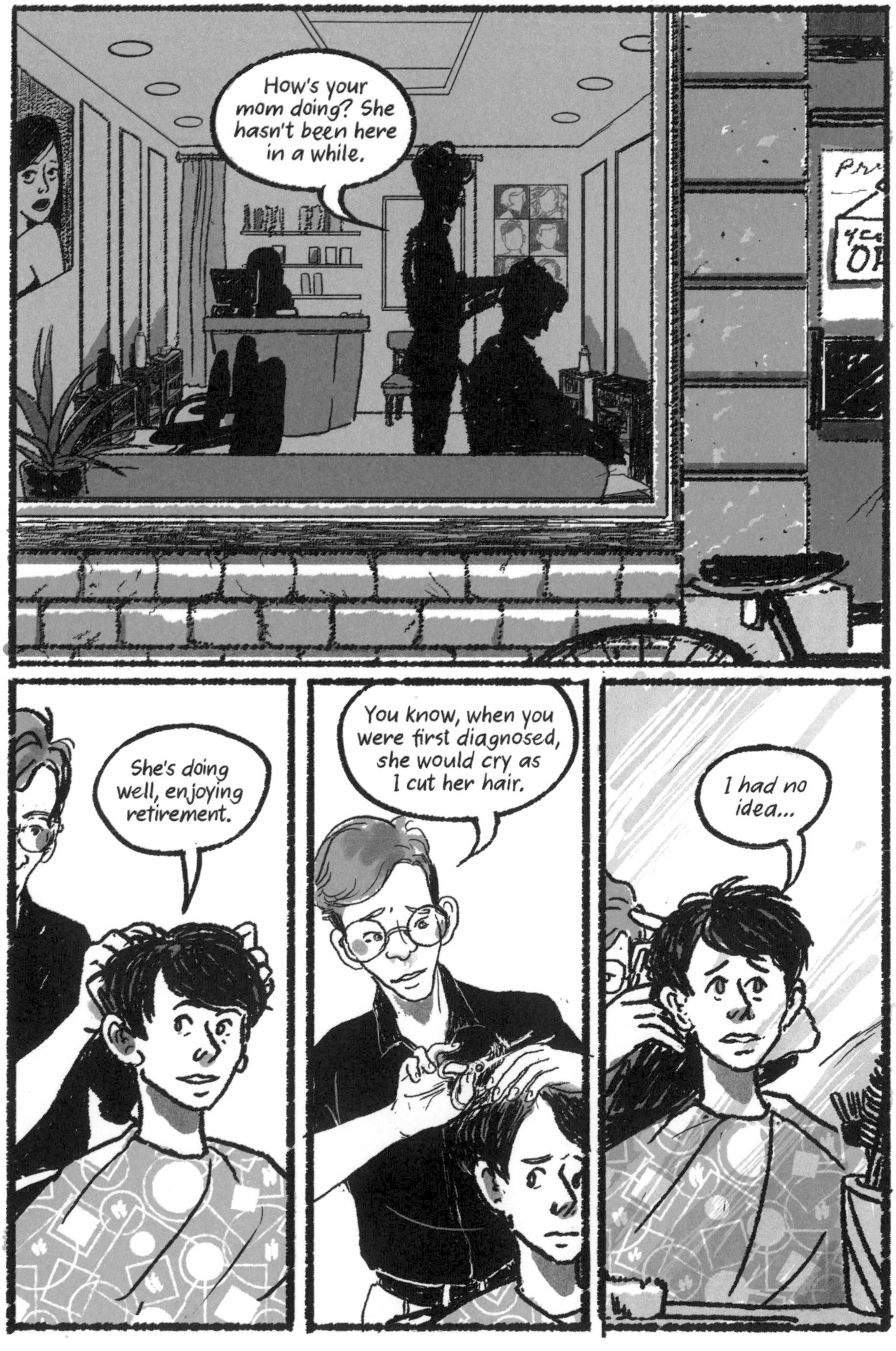
How's your mom doing? She hasn't been here in a while.
She's doing well, enjoying retirement.
You know, when you were first diagnosed, she would cry as I cut her hair.
I had no idea...

EPILOGUE

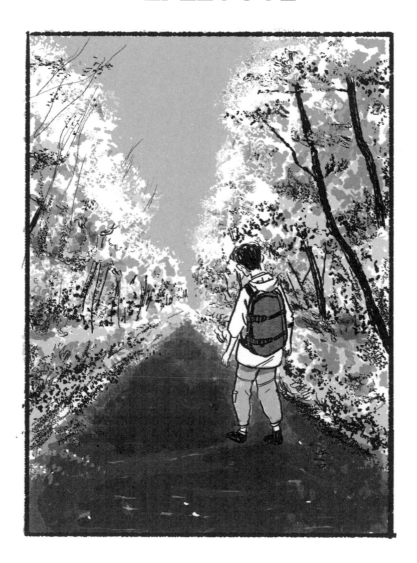

Cancer reshaped a lot of things in my life and brought on new fears.

I worry about recurrence and the effects of the drugs.

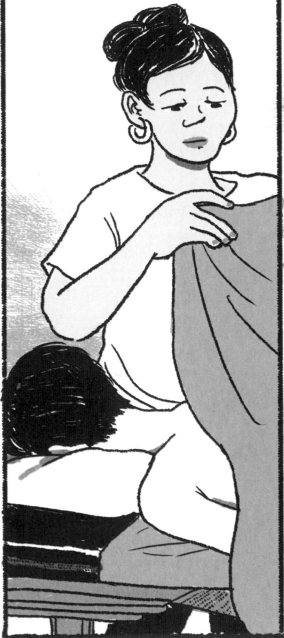

Without estrogen, the same cancer shouldn't come back, but without knowing why I got it in the first place, my doctors can't be sure. Plus, even though I already got one type of breast cancer, I still have the same (high) likelihood as anyone else of getting another type of breast cancer.

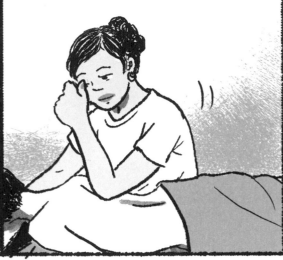

I wish getting it young meant that I'd paid my dues and was less likely to get it again.

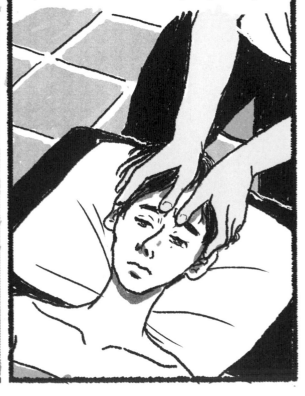

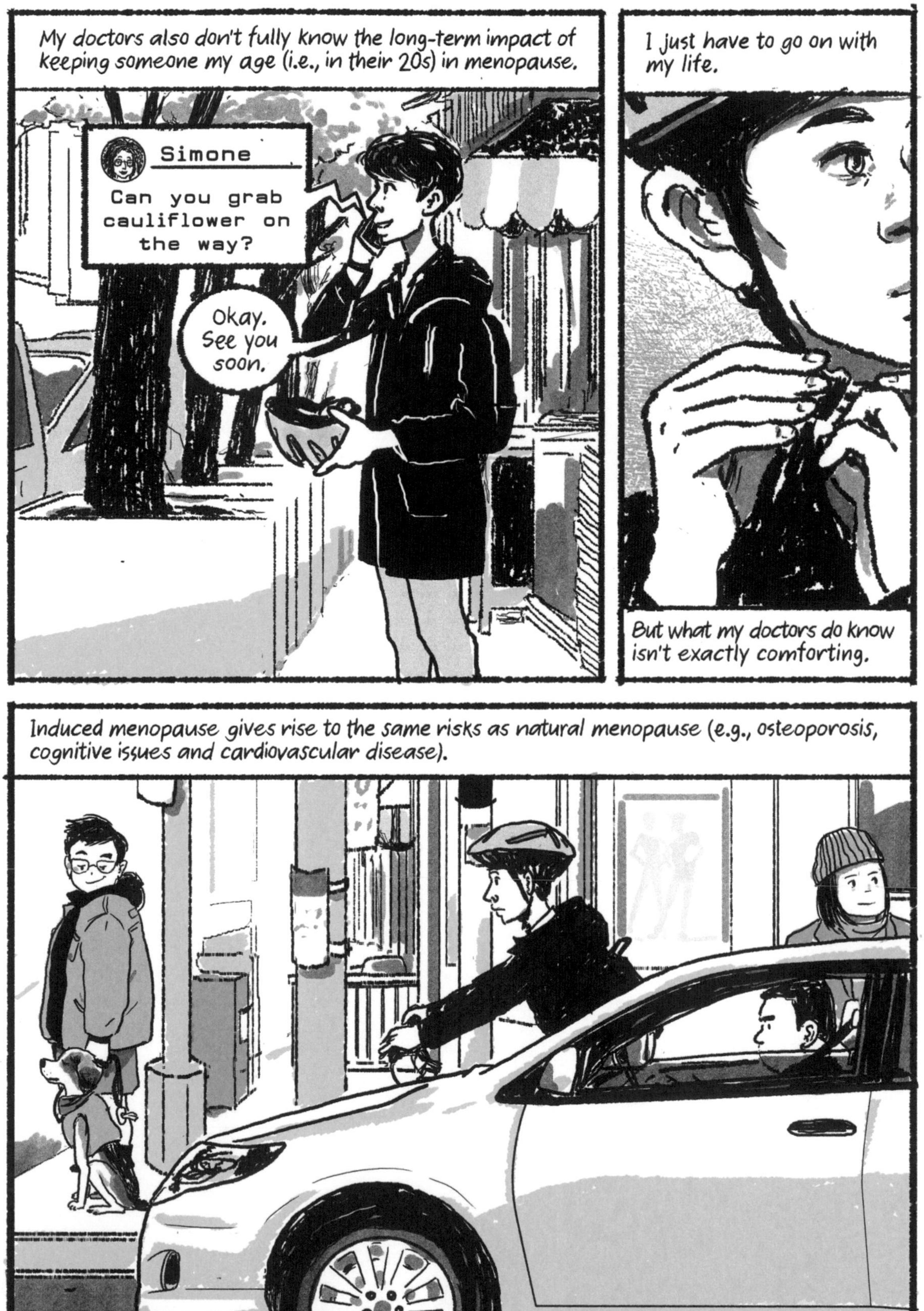
My doctors also don't fully know the long-term impact of keeping someone my age (i.e., in their 20s) in menopause.
Simone
Can you grab cauliflower on the way?
Okay. See you soon.
I just have to go on with my life.
But what my doctors do know isn't exactly comforting.
Induced menopause gives rise to the same risks as natural menopause (e.g., osteoporosis, cognitive issues and cardiovascular disease).

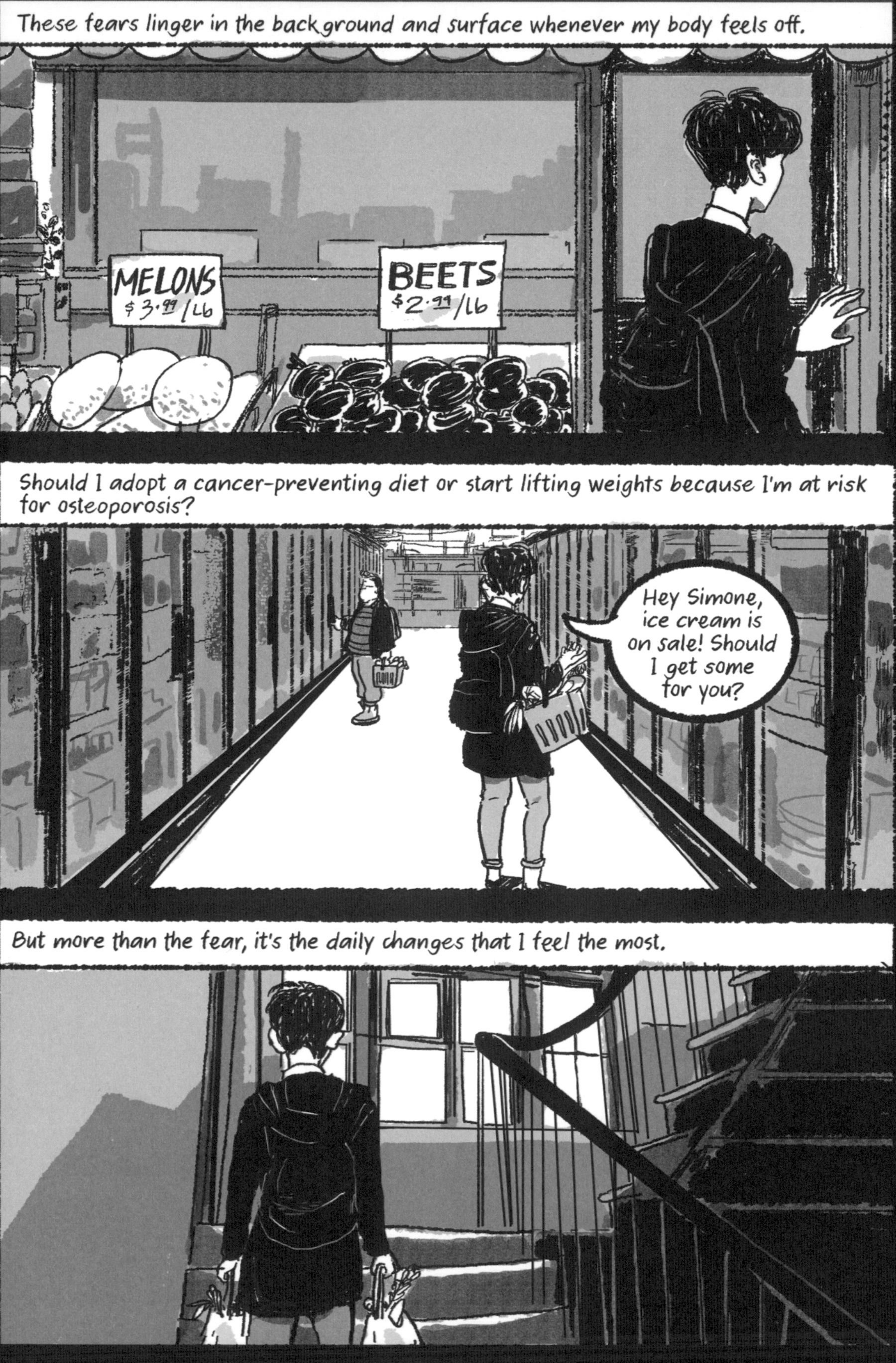
These fears linger in the background and surface whenever my body feels off.
MELONS $3.99/lb
BEETS $2.99/lb
Should I adopt a cancer-preventing diet or start lifting weights because I'm at risk for osteoporosis?
Hey Simone, ice cream is on sale! Should I get some for you?
But more than the fear, it's the daily changes that I feel the most.

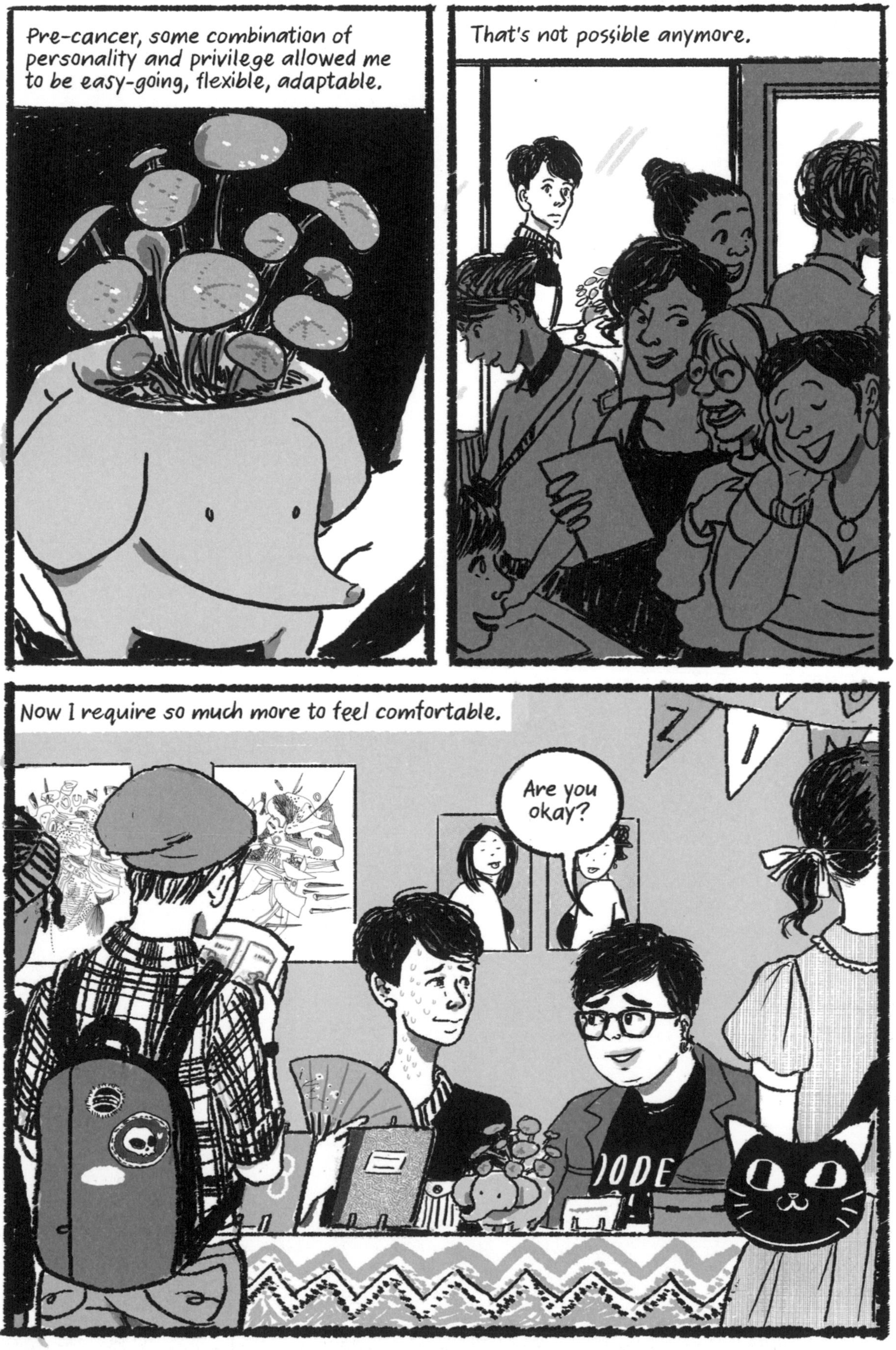
Pre-cancer, some combination of personality and privilege allowed me to be easy-going, flexible, adaptable.
That's not possible anymore.
Now I require so much more to feel comfortable.
Are you okay?

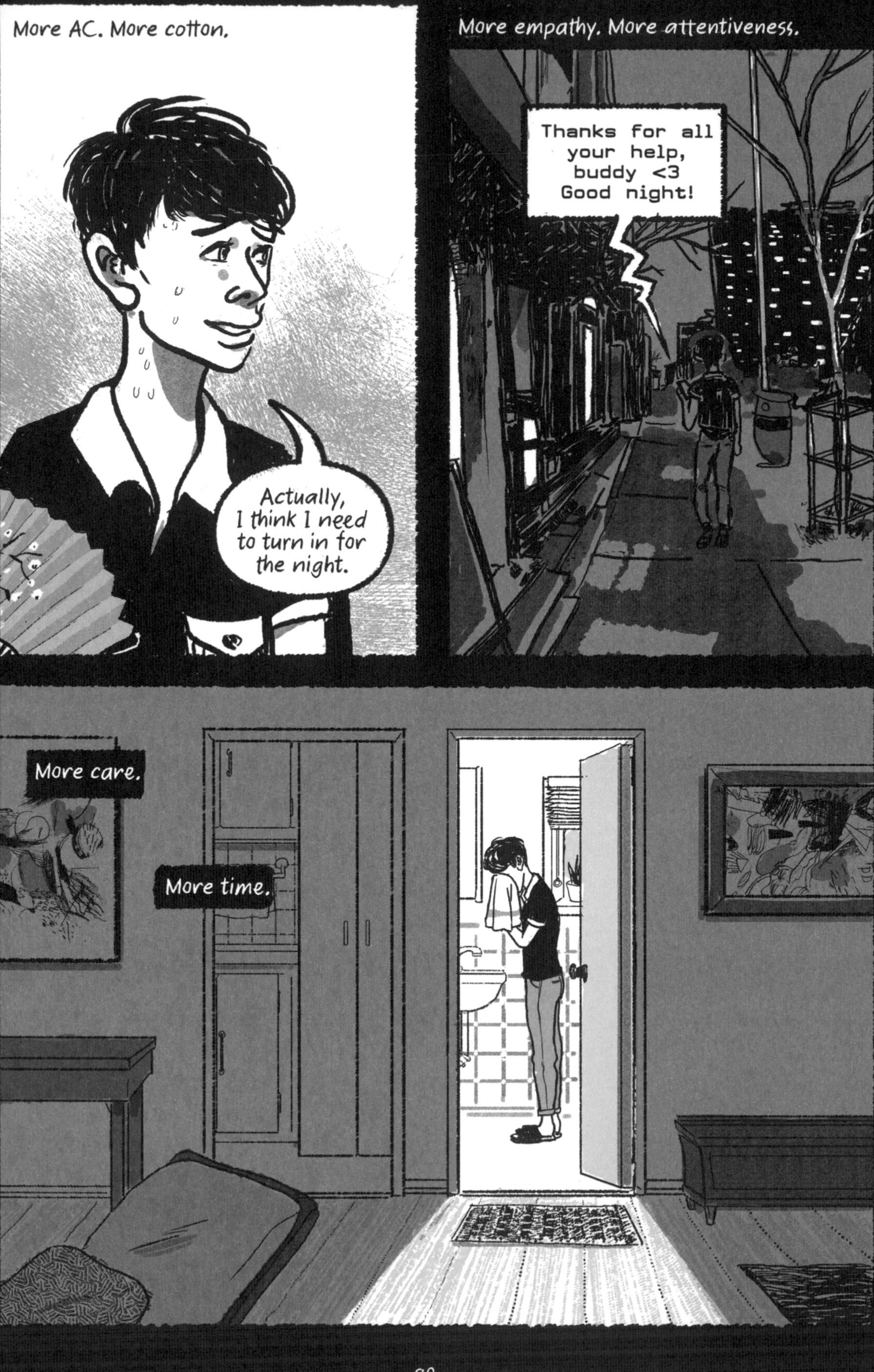
More AC. More cotton.
Actually, I think I need to turn in for the night.
More empathy. More attentiveness.
Thanks for all your help, buddy <3 Good night!
More care.
More time.

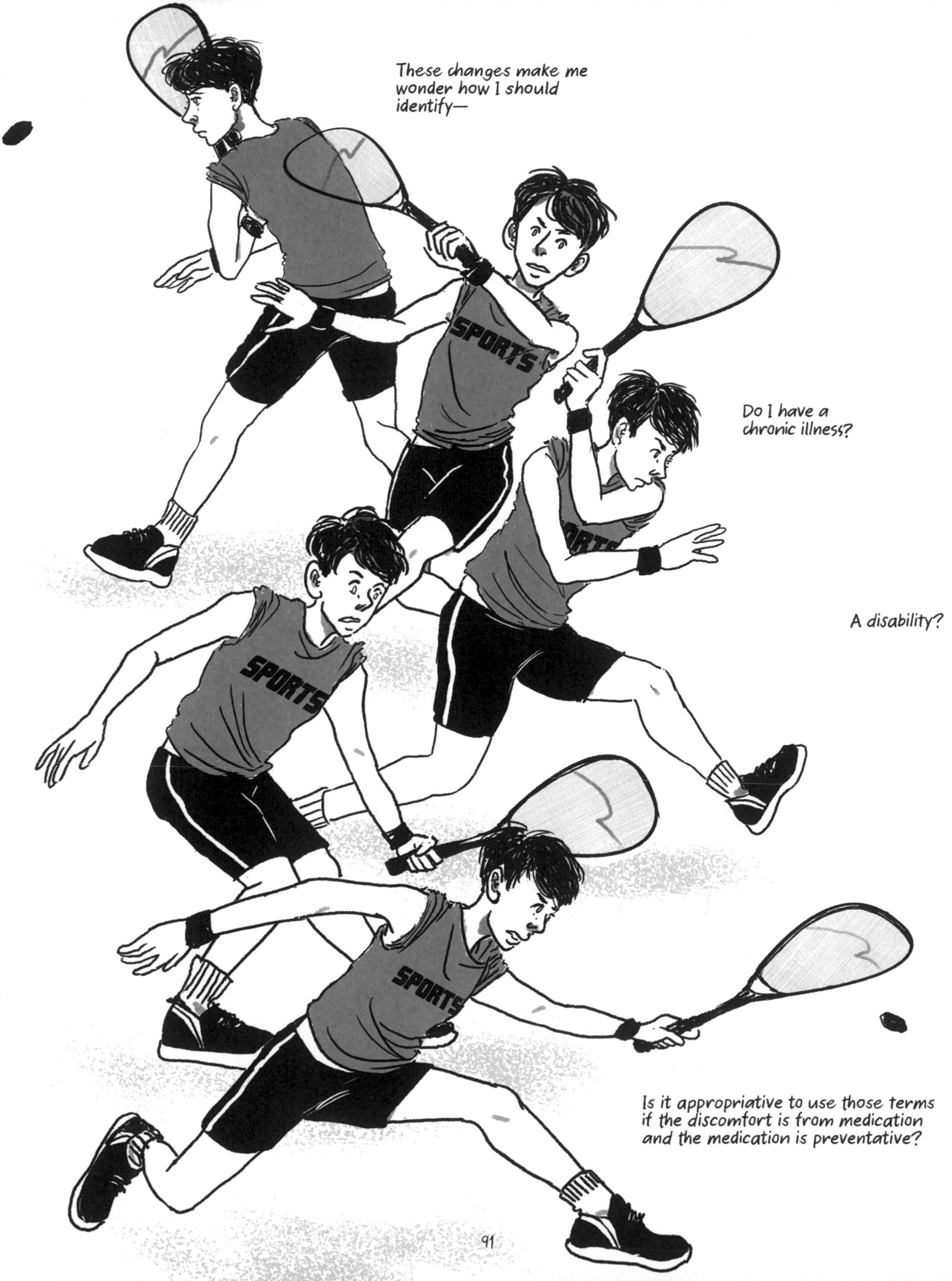
These changes make me wonder how I should identify—
Do I have a chronic illness?
A disability?
Is it appropriative to use those terms if the discomfort is from medication and the medication is preventative?
SPORTS
SPORTS
SPORTS

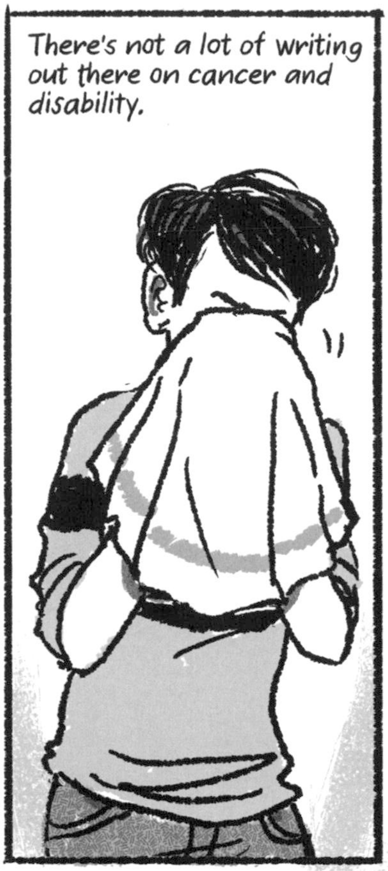
There's not a lot of writing out there on cancer and disability.

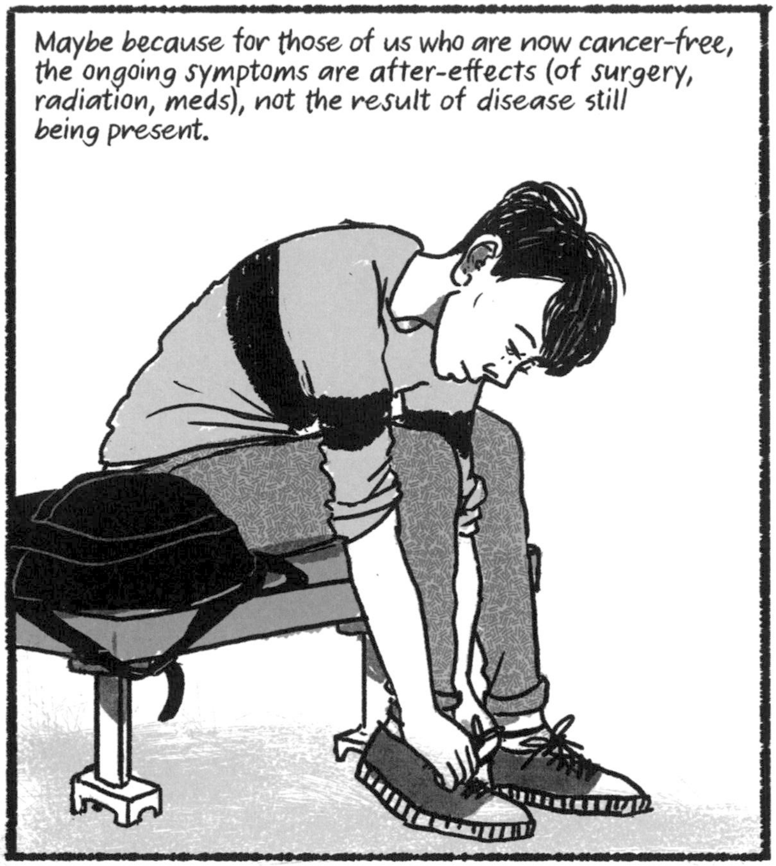
Maybe because for those of us who are now cancer-free, the ongoing symptoms are after-effects (of surgery, radiation, meds), not the result of disease still being present.

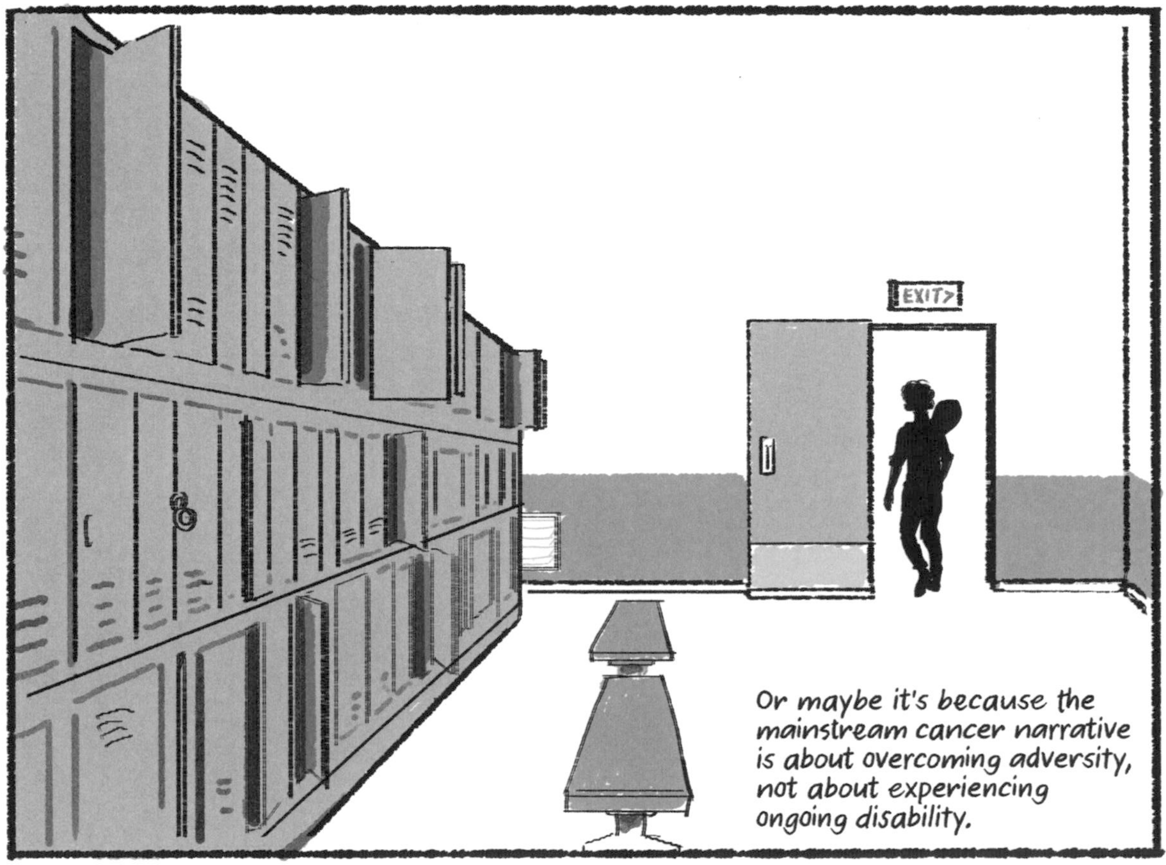
EXIT
Or maybe it's because the mainstream cancer narrative is about overcoming adversity, not about experiencing ongoing disability.

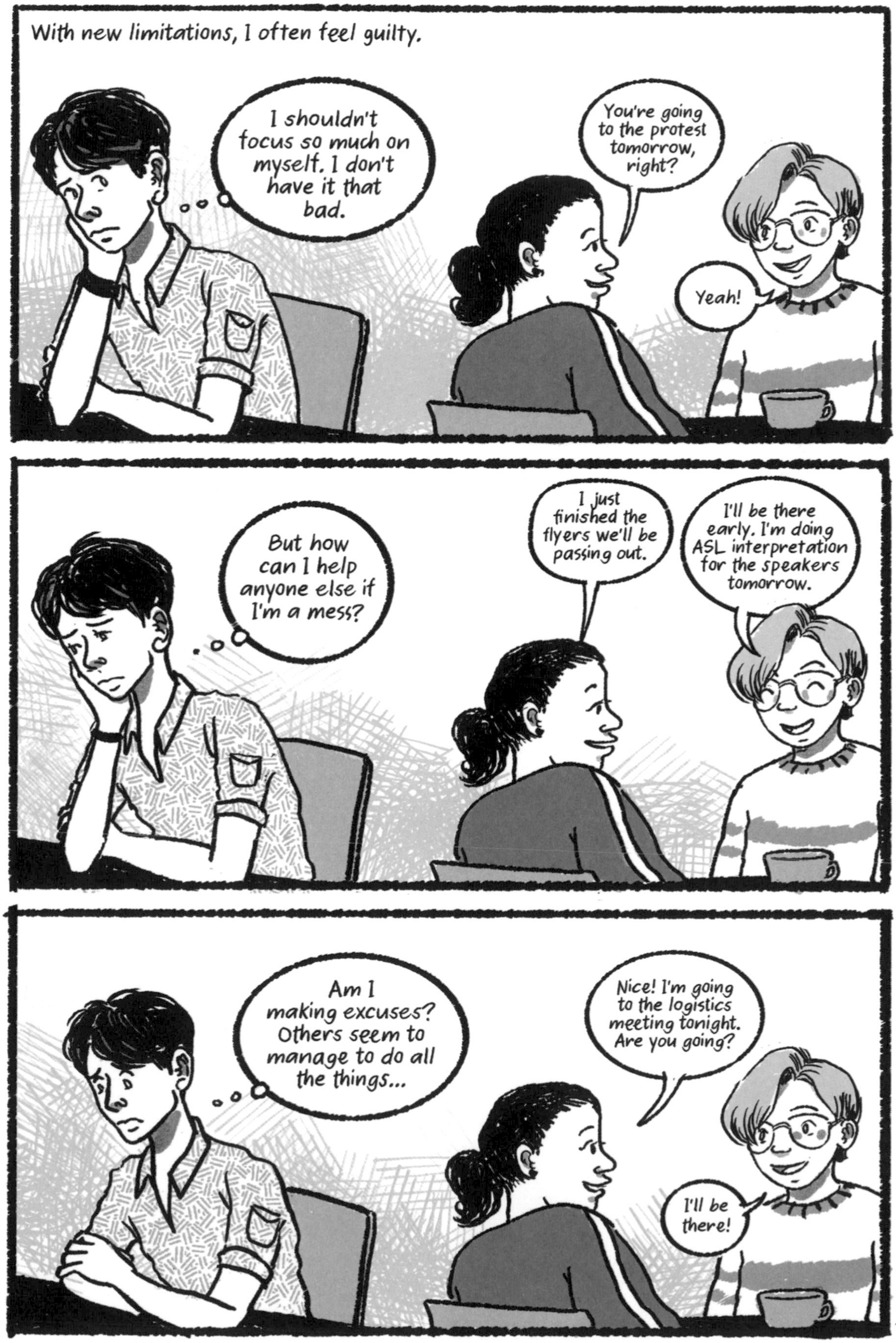
With new limitations, I often feel guilty.
I shouldn't focus so much on myself. I don't have it that bad.
You're going to the protest tomorrow, right?
Yeah!
But how can I help anyone else if I'm a mess?
I just finished the flyers we'll be passing out.
I'll be there early. I'm doing ASL interpretation for the speakers tomorrow.
Am I making excuses? Others seem to manage to do all the things...
Nice! I'm going to the logistics meeting tonight. Are you going?
I'll be there!

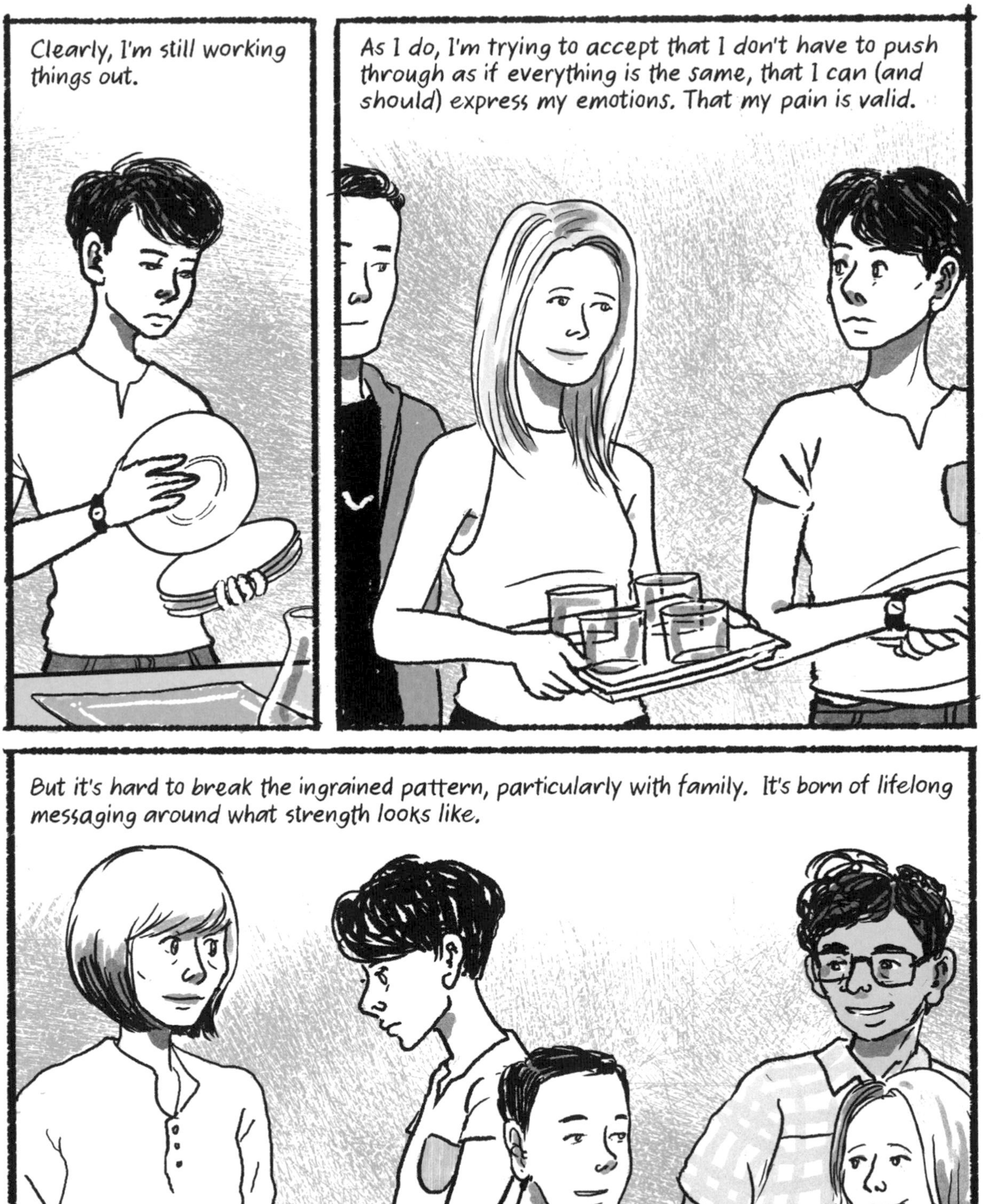
Clearly, I'm still working things out.
As I do, I'm trying to accept that I don't have to push through as if everything is the same, that I can (and should) express my emotions. That my pain is valid.
But it's hard to break the ingrained pattern, particularly with family. It's born of lifelong messaging around what strength looks like.

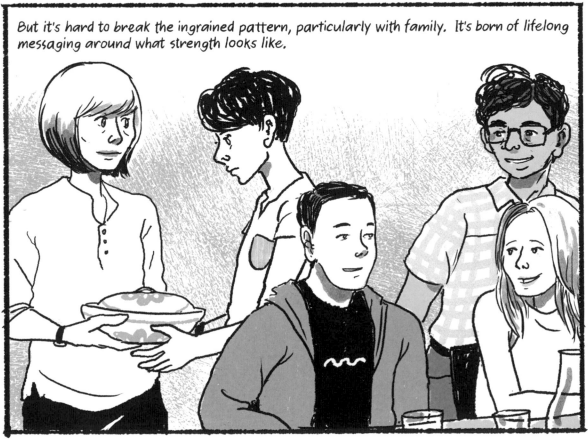

But I'm learning.
Learning to be deliberate with my energy.

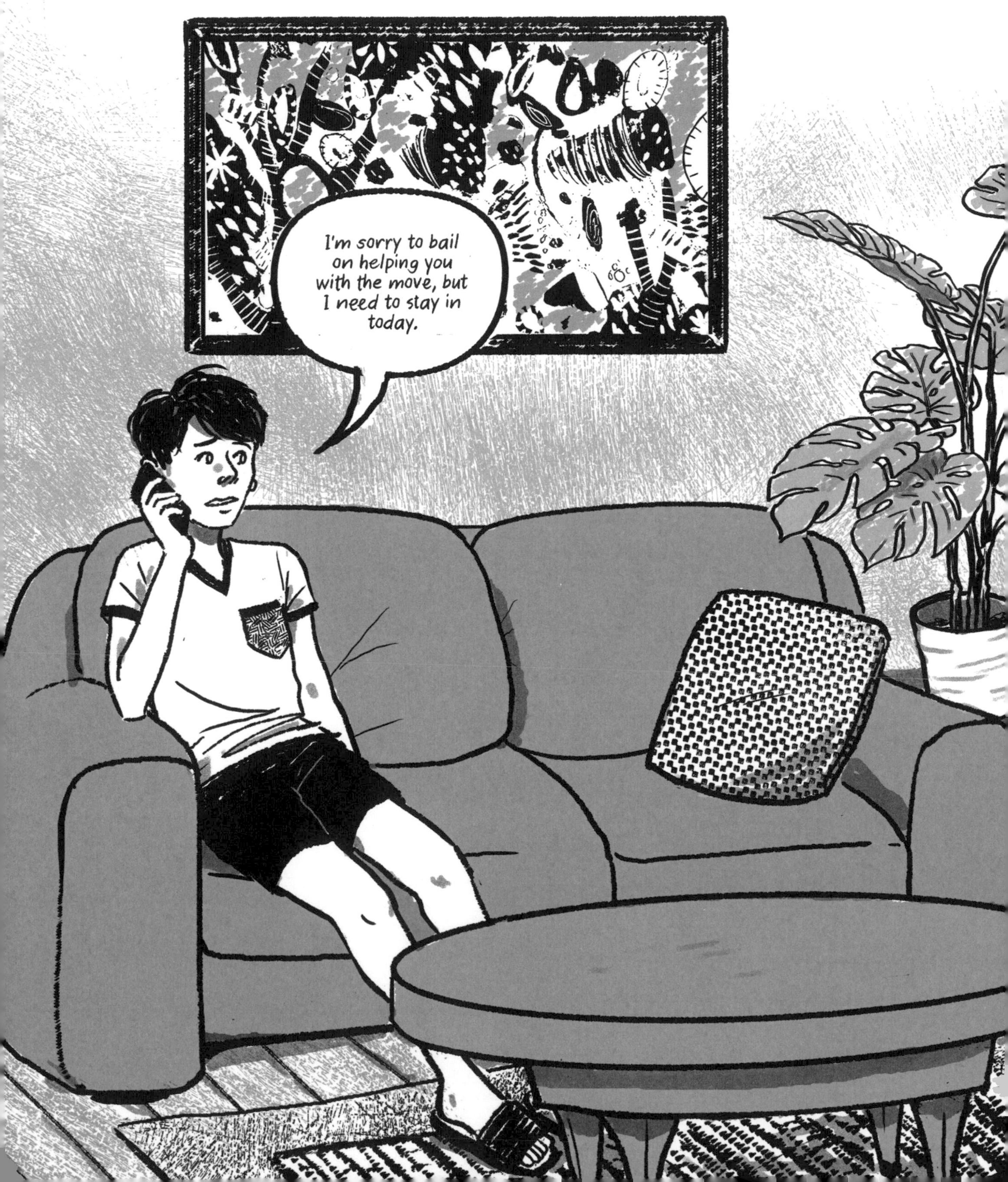
I'm sorry to bail on helping you with the move, but I need to stay in today.

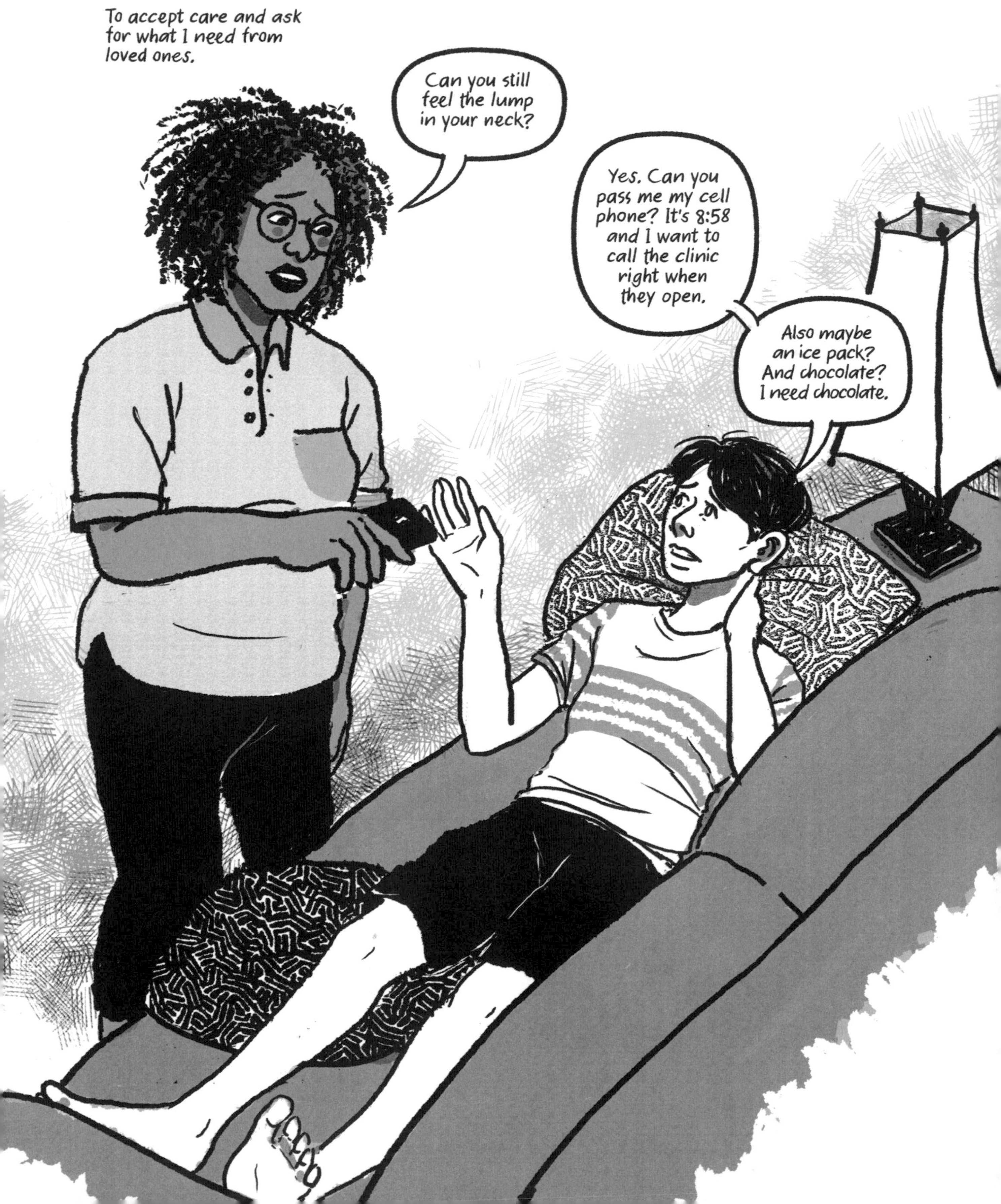
To accept care and ask for what I need from loved ones.
Can you still feel the lump in your neck?
Yes. Can you pass me my cell phone? It's 8:58 and I want to call the clinic right when they open.
Also maybe an ice pack? And chocolate? I need chocolate.

To do so even when I feel awkward.

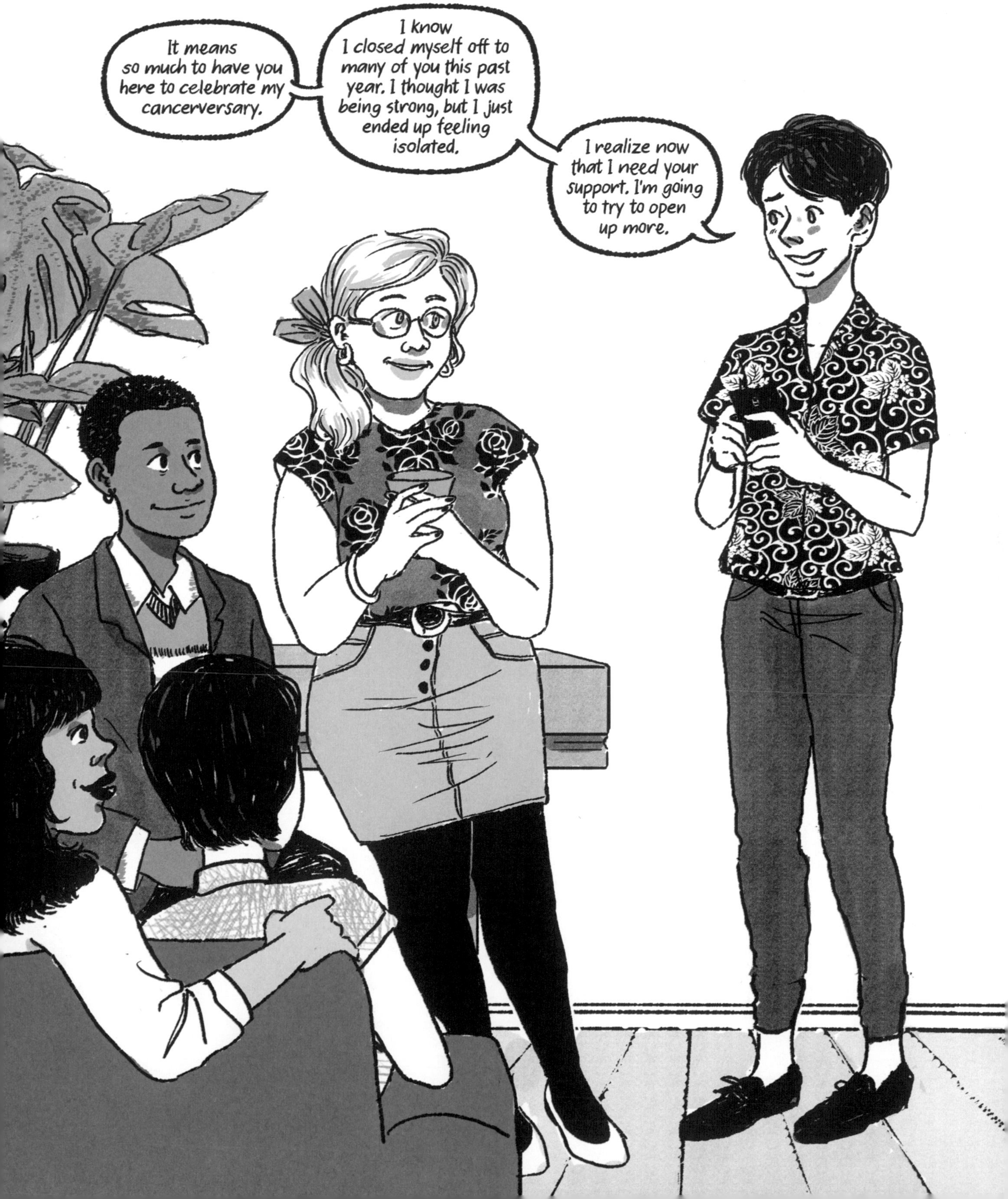
It means so much to have you here to celebrate my cancerversary.
I know I closed myself off to many of you this past year. I thought I was being strong, but I just ended up feeling isolated.
I realize now that I need your support. I'm going to try to open up more.

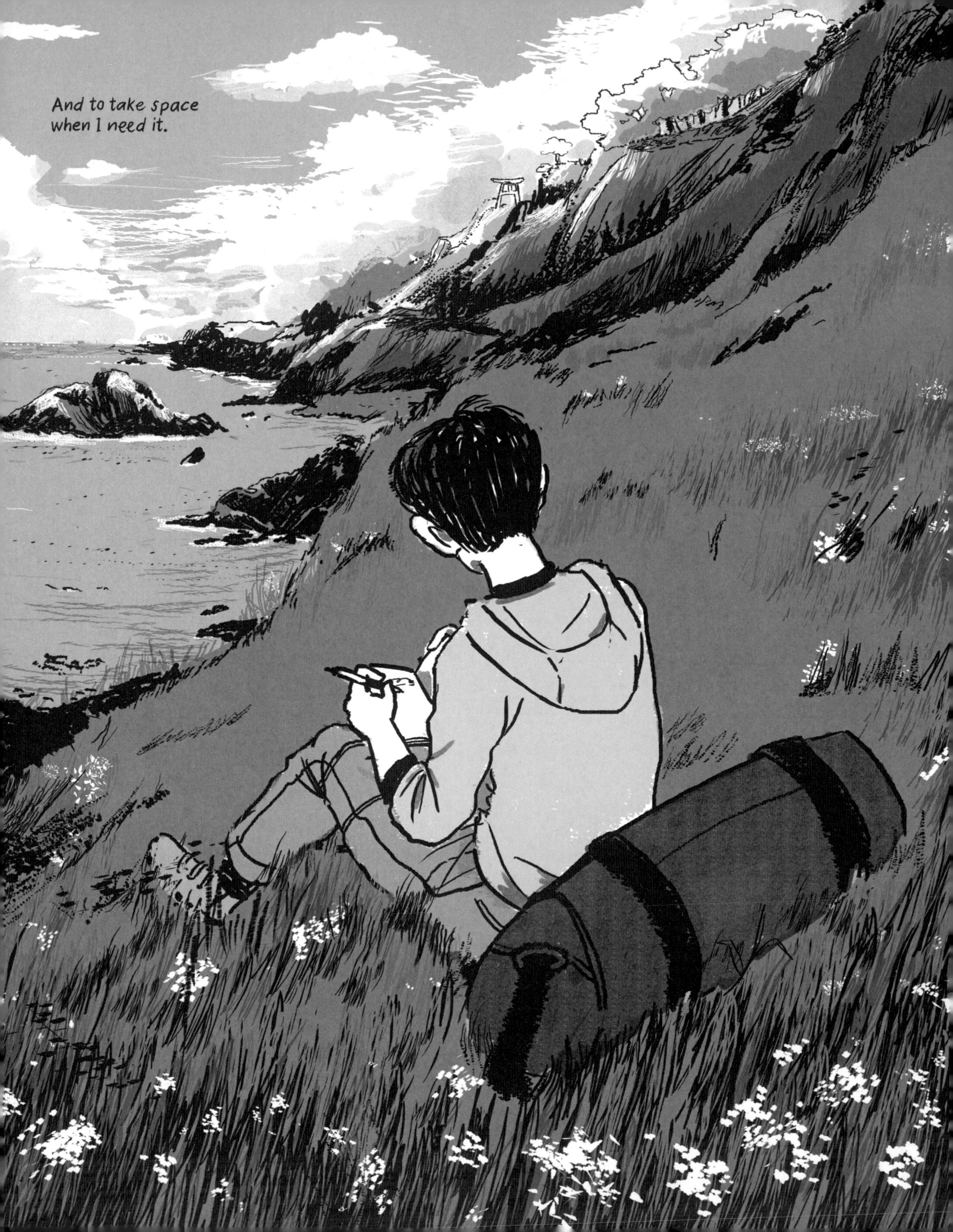
And to take space
when I need it.

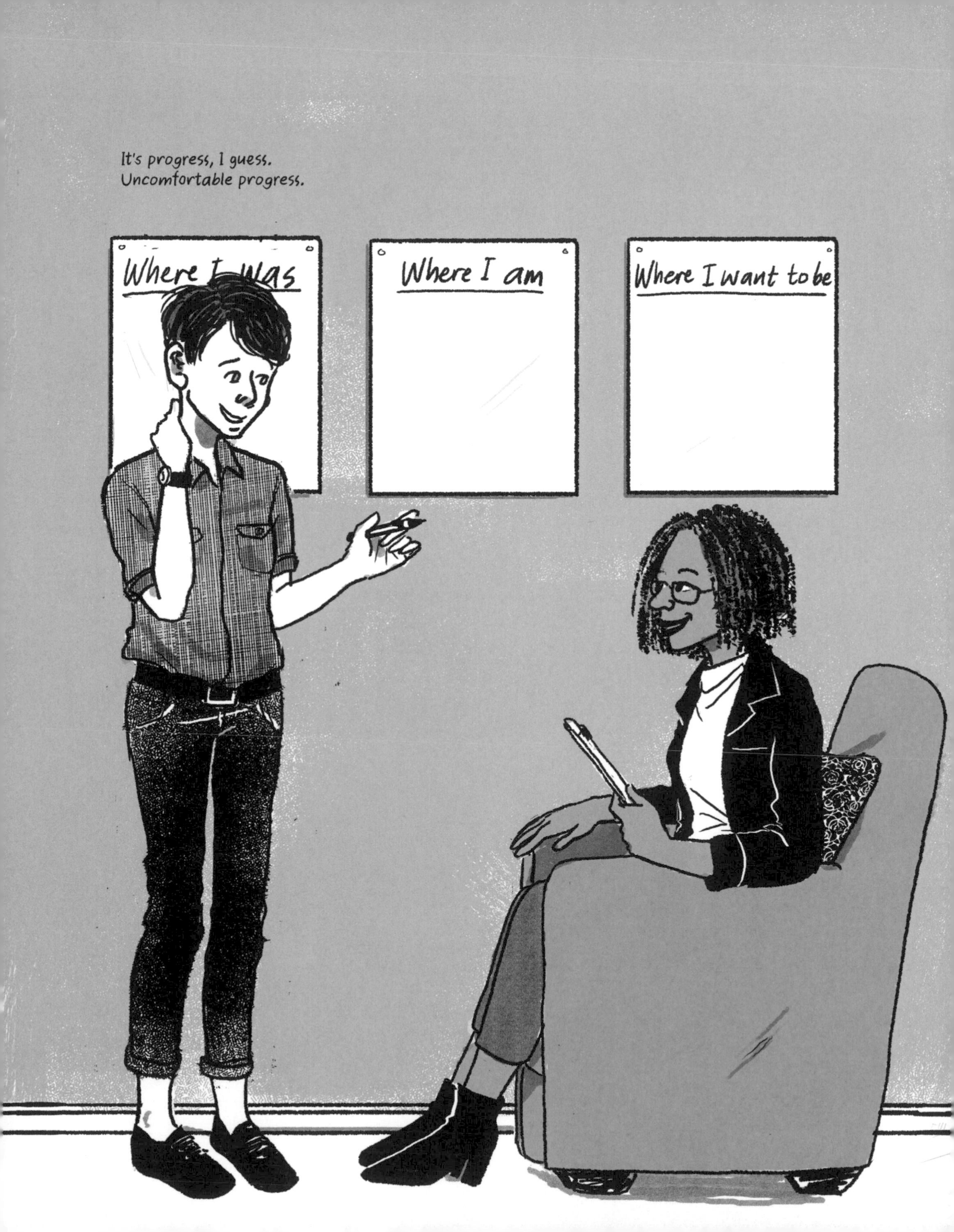
It's progress, I guess.
Uncomfortable progress.
Where I was
Where I am
Where I want to be

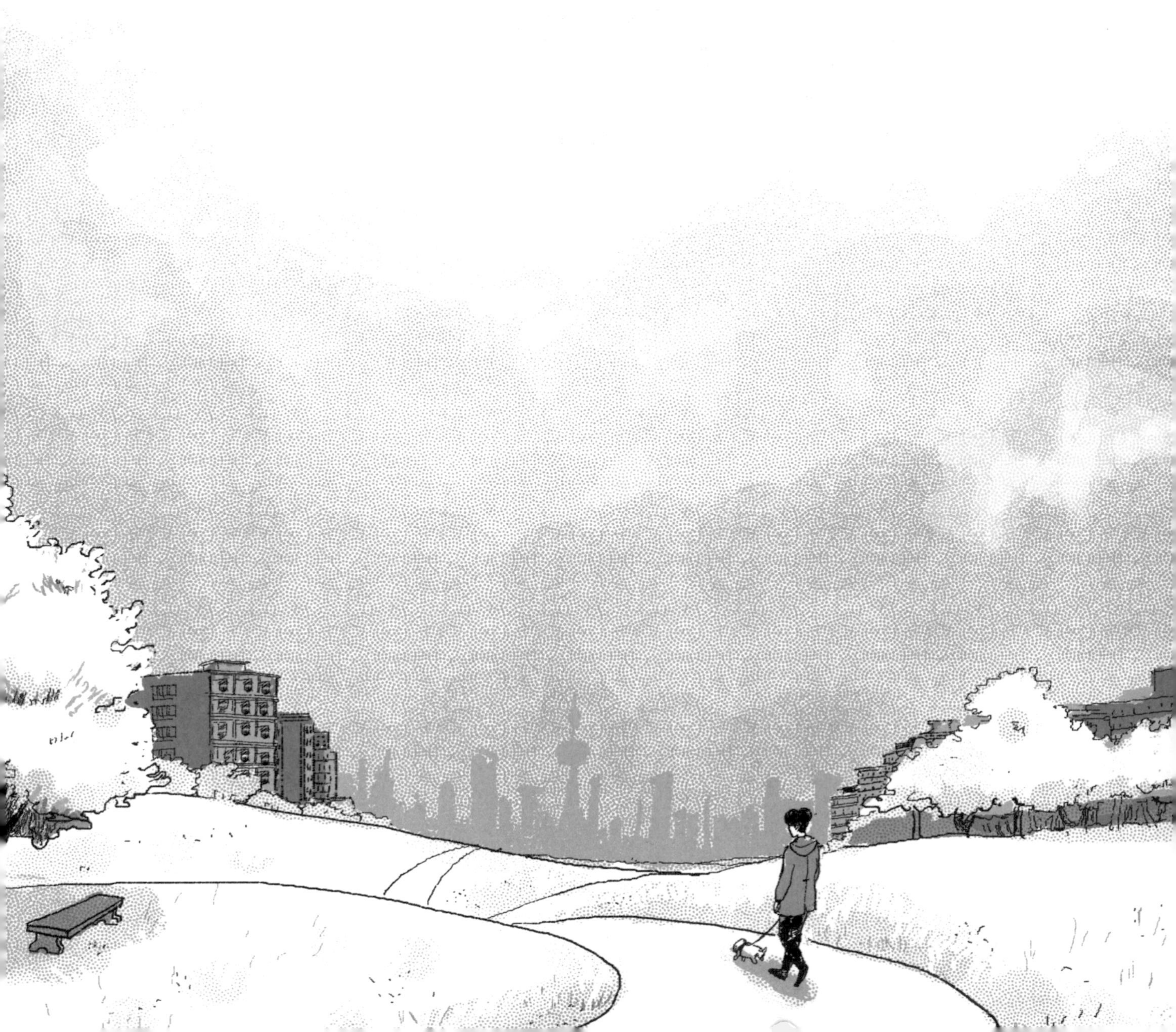

AFTERWORD

I'm not a big fan of the common sentiment, "Cancer made me a better person." I guess I tend to think that it shouldn't take a near-death experience to kick-start the desire to be a good person— to have balanced priorities, to live with passion, to be empathetic.

But then, cancer did make me a better person. Or at least, cancer triggered several practical changes that made me a better person.

For one, cancer led me to therapy, and therapy changed so much of how I relate to people, process emotions and plan my life.

Cancer was also the impetus for reducing my workweek to 4 days. A change that opened up time for me to focus on myself.

And of course, cancer put me on the path to writing this book. And this book, among many other changes, encouraged exploratory conversations with my family and helped me find a creativity I didn't know was there.

So, yes, cancer shook things up. But you won't find me living every day as if it's my last—that just seems exhausting! (Plus, what would happen to the revolution if we all operated that way?)

I recognize, though, that I'm lucky to very likely have many more days left to live. And I hope to use those days wisely (most of the time).

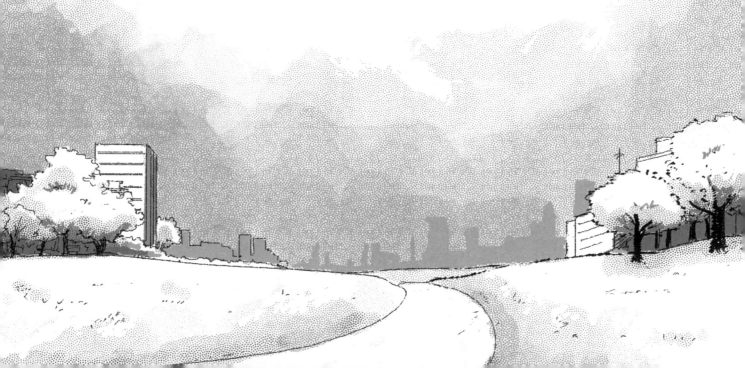

ACKNOWLEDGMENTS

There are so many people here now, and who have passed, for whom we are eternally grateful.

THIS STORY AND OUR COLLABORATION COULD NOT HAVE HAPPENED WITHOUT:
Audre Lorde, who wrote a version of this book long before us; Michelle Campos, who was instrumental in connecting Kimiko and Keet; Kendra Boileau, for her insightful feedback; and the Graphic Medicine folks, who showed us there was a community out there for this type of work.

This story came alive with the skilful edits early on from Tara-Michelle Ziniuk and the amazing support of the Arsenal Pulp Press team. We are immensely thankful.

ADDITIONAL THANKS FROM KIMIKO TO:
Ayaan, for nurturing the seeds of creativity before anyone else; Simone, for her keen eye and encouragement to keep at it; Nadha, for understanding the journey and providing thoughtful input; Jenny, for her love and joy and care; Joan, for her guidance throughout; and my parents, for cradling me back to health and embracing this story, even when it came with difficult conversations.

And Keet: I will be forever grateful. Your masterful craft turned this book into a work of art beyond my wildest dreams.

KEET WOULD ALSO LIKE TO THANK:
Kimiko, for her trust and generosity throughout the building of this book. Much love and gratitude.

Althea, Lorraine, Sukie, Phil, Gillian, Andrew, Sves, Eloisa, Mary, CJ, CB, Jo, Alyos, Emily, Jenelle, Addie, Teresa, Lynn and everyone who celebrated, commiserated, encouraged and supported me in a myriad of immeasurable ways and kept me going.

Tita Ninang and Tita Baby, whose love, labour and delicious foods are a cornerstone in the making of this book.

My mother, Bettina, and my siblings, Ezra and Ken, for being a stronghold of love and support. Mahal ko kayo.

Sa aking mga ninuno. Ito po'y isang maliit na handog para sa inyo. Mula sa kaibuturan ng aking puso't pagkatao, maraming salamat.

And lastly, thanks to our doggos, because, well, points for being cute, right? To everyone, thank you, thank you, thank you.

—Kimiko and Keet

Photo credit: Jenny Vasquez

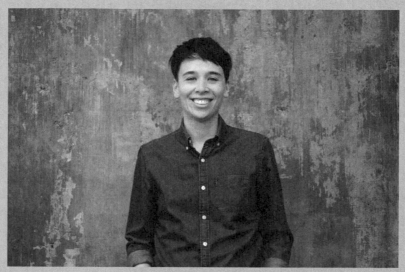

KIMIKO TOBIMATSU is an employment and human rights lawyer by day. *Kimiko Does Cancer* is her first book.
kimikodoescancer.com

Photo credit: Eloisa Guerrero

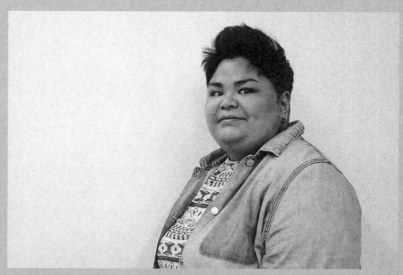

KEET GENIZA is an illustrator and comic artist. Born and raised in Manila, she moved to Toronto in 2006 and has since immersed herself in zines and comics as a way to document her struggles as a queer immigrant woman of colour. *Kimiko Does Cancer* is her first book.
makeshiftlove.com